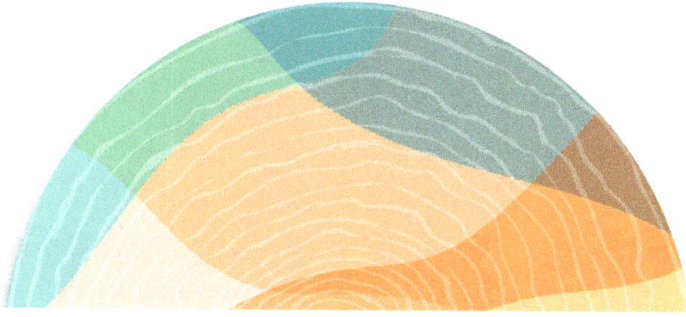

Gerontological Care and Reflective Practice

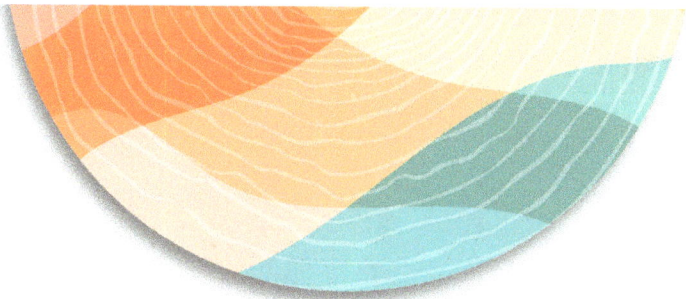

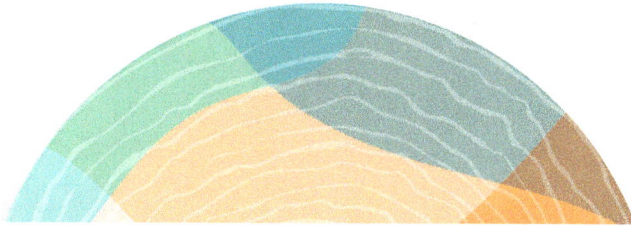

Gerontological Care and Reflective Practice

Person-Centered and Caring Dimensions

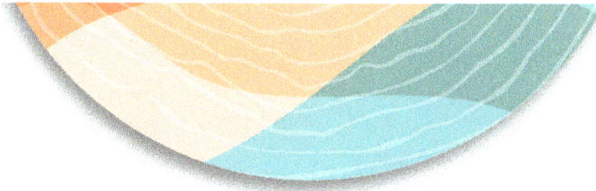

OLIVIA CATOLICO
Dominican University of California

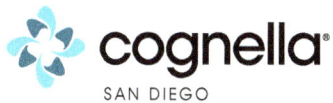

cognella®
SAN DIEGO

Bassim Hamadeh, CEO and Publisher
Amanda Martin, Executive Publisher
Zoe Flores, Project Editor
Casey Hands, Senior Production Editor
Jess Estrella, Senior Graphic Designer
JoHannah McDonald, Licensing Coordinator
Monica O'Keefe, Editoral Associate
Natalie Piccotti, Director of Marketing
Kassie Graves, Senior Vice President, Editorial
Alia Bales, Director, Project Editorial and Production

cognella | ACADEMIC PUBLISHING
320 South Cedros Ave., Ste. 400, Solana Beach, CA 92075

BRIEF CONTENTS

DETAILED CONTENTS

PREFACE

This book evolved out of observations of the escalating "medicalization" of aging instead of the humanity of aging. Authentic caring and honest introspection about one's practice and meaningful relationship to older adults has diminished. This, perhaps, provides the seedlings of stigma and exclusion, which are socially embedded in health care systems.

This book was also developed out of a growing realization that there is little attention given to older adults and the fact that we are all aging. The United Nations has elevated the significance of aging as a global phenomenon by declaring 2021–2030 as the *Decade of Healthy Aging*. Within my own professional networks and among my faculty peers, few are aware of this as the mid-decade point quickly approaches.

For critics who may see this book as superficial and not comprehensive enough about the care of older persons, note that there are a plethora of textbooks about the pathophysiology of aging and the medical and pharmacological treatment and management of chronic diseases.

Important premises upon which the scope of this book is based are that:

- A person-centered relationship that respects the uniqueness of each individual is essential to effective care.

- Older adults possess capability and capacity to learn, process, and utilize new knowledge, information, and skills.

- Older adults have rich, varied, diverse, and unique life experiences that inform their worldview.

- Older adults are capable of maintaining wellness and quality of life as they age.

Given the above, this book is a distinct exploration and overview of the social context in which aging occurs. The reader peers into social determinants of health, health care disparities, migration, and aging, combating ageism, and advocacy for older adults. Questions, case studies, journal articles, and internet resources to facilitate further inquiry, deeper exploration of issues, and praxis are accentuated throughout the book. The faculty may choose to use these resources in a manner befitting faculty goals, the learner's needs, or level of study.

While the book is not written from a particular perspective, for the sake of transparency, the author has lived and worked among immigrant, migrant, and refugee communities in the U.S. and has served abroad in a health care capacity in Uganda, Tanzania, and Costa Rica. It is my hope and open invitation that the book will also be used in global communities and other programs that prepare health care workers to elevate the status of older adults and promote successful aging in place.

LOOKING INWARD: REFLECTIVE PRACTICE

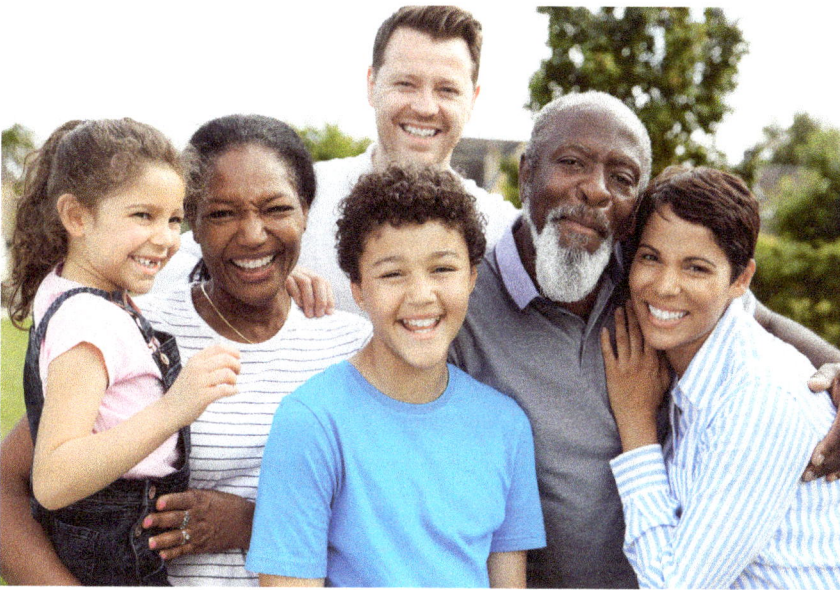

Image 1.1

Overview

This chapter centers the learner with a foundational perspective toward care of the older adult and identifies core professional values essential for reflective practice. Professional values are grounded in a code of ethics and guide practice. Nursing and caring for older adults requires certain knowledge, skills, competencies, and also that one cultivates and engages in reflective practice. This chapter also identifies assumptions about older adults upon which this book is based.

Outcomes

The learner:

1. Articulates the Code of Ethics and its relationship to professional practice

2. Reflects upon one's own core values of caring practice

3. Describes social determinants of health that influence the quality of care of older adults

Affirming Assumptions

Myths, stereotypes, and misinformation about older adults and aging perpetuate falsities, bias, discrimination, and health care inequalities. Furthermore, belief in these notions may deter access to care and a universal right to be healthy. This book is founded on key assumptions, in which older adults

1. experience aging as a personal and individualized life process accompanied by normal physiological changes.

2. can continue to lead a full quality of life, with optimum health and function.

3. have the capacity and choice to make informed health and end-of-life decisions based on reliable and valid scientific evidence, as well as personal preferences.

4. have unique and diverse life experiences, which have shaped their beliefs, values, and actions about health and well-being.

5. have acquired a lifetime of knowledge and skills to serve as effective mentors to others.

6. have the capacity to learn and acquire new knowledge, skills, and to utilize this information in everyday living for better health.

7. flourish in an environment that meets basic needs; promotes health and provides ready access to health care; provides social support (affect, affirmation, and aid); facilitates community participation; and values their voices and contributions to society.

Given these stated assumptions, nurses have a professional obligation to self, older adults entrusted to their care, and the broader community.

The Groundwork for Professional Practice: Self-Reflection and Reflective Practice "Praxis"

The rapid evolution and advancement of technology has its advantages and disadvantages. Technological applications can be employed across various health care disciplines and in many spheres daily of life. They can also present an invasive bombardment of external sensory stimuli influencing beliefs on how one should appear, act, feel, think, and behave. This distraction takes away moments of true engagement alone with oneself.

Self-reflection invites internal self-dialogue, awareness, mindfulness, and personal evaluation of one's actions. It cultivates receptivity to new ideas and may ultimately lead to intentional change in one's actions and professional practice. Through self-reflection, one may see the personal perspective within the broader circle of one's professional influence. Having this broader view may facilitate sustainable change that benefits self, professional practice, and bringing about effective health outcomes for older adults.

Looking inward upon oneself requires courage, humility, resilience, and an acceptance and openness to learning and discovery. Listening to a reflective internal dialogue can be challenging in the face of external demands, roles, and responsibilities. It is natural to brush off perceptions of negativity, whether from family, friends, coworkers, or supervisors, who offer helpful attempts in the form of corrective actions, performance evaluations, or advice.

Self-reflection allows one the space and silence to acknowledge one's strengths, limitations, and appreciation of the unique identity and values that one brings to professional practice. One may ask, "To what extent does care, respect, and dignity extend to self? Others?" The American Nurses Association (ANA, 2015) Code of Ethics[1], Provision 5, clearly affirms the importance of duty to self and duty to others. The ability to care for others effectively with compassion and empathy, while grounded in an evidence-based practice, requires rejuvenation of mind, body, and spirit.

Reflective Practice, "Praxis"

Looking inward facilitates the cultivation of "praxis" or reflective practice. Praxis is "The action and reflection of people upon their world in order to transform it," as aptly defined by the educator philosopher, Paulo Freire (1970) in his initial work. As a caring profession, the work of nursing seeks to transform the health and well-being of others. This transformation extends to persons, families, groups, communities, and the social structures built by humans in service of others. Underlying praxis is a critical consciousness that is vital to transformative change, whereby nurses are held accountable for competent actions and decision-making in care and also

---

1   **Note from the Publisher:** This book references the 2015 edition of the American Nurses Association (ANA) Code of Ethics. An updated version was released on January 29, 2025. We recommend readers refer to the latest code for up-to-date guidelines. For more details, please visit the ANA's website at https://codeofethics.ana.org/provisions

ongoing examination of systems, microsystems, power structures, and dynamics for the intentional purposes of improving the quality of care for older adults.

Nursing has long since embraced Freire's philosophy of praxis, and this is echoed in the advocacy work of nursing scholars, researchers, and practitioners. Embodied in *nursing praxis* are concepts that describe multiple patterns of knowing that form the basis of nursing knowledge. These are emancipatory (social justice), ethical (right and wrong), personal (awareness of self and others), aesthetic (meaning and intent), and empiric (how things work and knowing through sensory experiences). Emancipatory knowing requires awareness and critical reflection upon inequities that result in transformative interactions at the clinical or point-of-care patient encounter (Chinn et al., 2022).

Nursing praxis continues to be an important focal point within the profession (Fry et al., 2013; Hills et al., 2021; Kagan et al., 2009; Keith, 1987; Rafii et al., 2022; Rolfe, 2006). Nursing praxis is facilitated through awareness, reflection, and a sense of critical consciousness. Critical consciousness as a thought process questions the status quo about health and social systems. This inquiry leads to transformative action that is effective, meaningful, relevant, and sustainable. Nursing praxis is individual and collective. It is informed by a professional code of ethics and nursing knowledge acquired through emancipatory, ethical, personal, aesthetic, and empiric modes of learning.

Code of Ethics

Praxis by definition embodies social action and professional comportment. Social action refers to those collective, organized behaviors that address inequities. Professional comportment refers to the attributes of mutual respect, harmony, commitment, and collaboration for which the individual nurse is responsible and accountable (Clickner & Shirey, 2013). These attributes are demonstrated through effective, respectful, and collaborative nurse-patient, nurse-nurse, and nurse–health care team interactions and communications. Furthermore, the American Nurses Association (ANA) Code of Ethics is a beacon integrating and illuminating social action, professional comportment, and practice (ANA, 2015). The learner is encouraged to fully explore the Code with interpretative statements (Fowler, 2015a). The Code, since its inception in 1950, reflects values of the profession, ideals, and commitments. Key provisions of the Code are detailed below (ANA, 2015):

Provision 1: The nurse practices with compassion and respect for the inherent dignity, worth, and unique attributes of every person.

Provision 2: The nurse's primary commitment is to the patient, whether an individual, family, group, community, or population.

Provision 3: The nurse promotes, advocates for, and protects the rights, health, and safety of the patient.

Provision 4: The nurse has authority, accountability, and responsibility for nursing practice; makes decisions; and takes actions consistent with the obligation to promote health and to provide optimal care.

Provision 5: The nurse owes the same duties to self as to others, including the responsibility to promote health and safety, preserve wholeness of character and integrity, maintain competence, and continue personal and professional growth.

Provision 6: The nurse, through individual and collective effort, establishes, maintains, and improves the ethical environment of the work setting and conditions of employment that are conducive to safe, quality health care.

Provision 7: The nurse, in all roles and settings, advances the profession through research and scholarly inquiry, professional standards development, and the generation of both nursing and health policy.

Provision 8: The nurse collaborates with other health professionals and the public to protect human rights, promote health diplomacy, and reduce health disparities.

Provision 9: The profession of nursing, collectively through its professional organizations, must articulate nursing values, maintain the integrity of the profession, and integrate principles of social justice into nursing and health policy.

The nurse has both a professional and a societal role, as illuminated in the Code of Ethics. Figure 1.1 depicts the relationship of nursing praxis and its influence upon the profession, health, and health care systems.

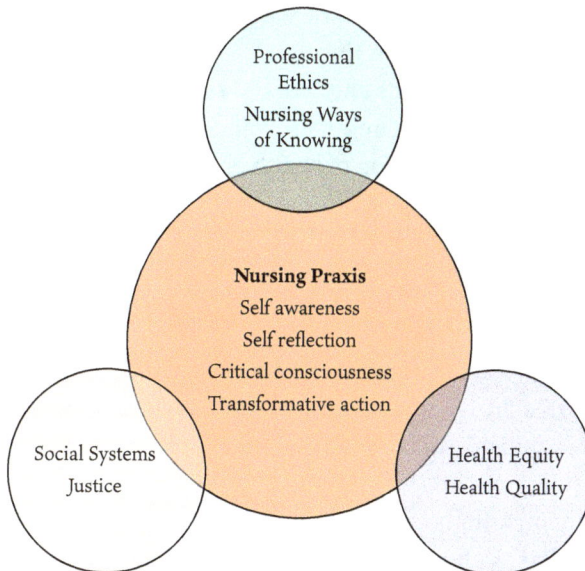

FIGURE 1.1   Relationship of Praxis, Ethics, and Knowing, Health, and Social Systems

Core Values of Caring Practices

Caring, dignity, health, respect, well-being, and worth are inherent values articulated in the code. These core values further extend to the relationship between the nursing profession and society as nursing's social contract in recognizing health needs and promoting public health.

On a personal level, one may have a personal mission statement that embodies individual knowledge, skills, abilities, and values. In practice, at the personal-transpersonal level, core values are demonstrated in one's verbal and nonverbal communication, behaviors, and interactions at the point-of-care encounter with patients, peer colleagues, and the interprofessional health care team. At the systems or organizational level, core values are communicated in mission and vision statements and are integrated throughout core processes policies and strategic plans of the organization. Actualization of values and caring practices are acknowledged in various ways. These may be through recognition of excellence, special achievement, or designation status. These may further be articulated in standards of gerontological nursing practice (ANA, 2019), standards of quality (USDHHS, n.d.-b) a bill of rights, and systems plans, and may be further evaluated through tangible means to determine the extent to which core values are lived.

The relationship between the profession and society is reflected in the ANA's social policy statement (Fowler, 2015b). A profession regulates its own practice, and therefore, standards of practice and competence are defined and described by professional organizations. Standards of practice range from generalist to specialty areas of practice. They define and describe caring service, knowledge, skills and competence, responsibility and accountability, progress and development, autonomy, and freedom to practice within the scope of one's educational preparation and competence.

The interrelationships between the code (ANA, 2015), nursing's social policy (Fowler, 2015b), and the standards and scope of practice (ANA, 2019) are essential to the integrity of the profession and its social contract. To expand further upon these interrelationships, a discussion of health ensues with attention to social determinants of health and health equity.

Health, Social Determinants, and Health Equity

Health is the optimum state of holistic well-being of individuals, families, groups, or communities. Nurses promote and facilitate optimum attainment of health. Health embodies physical, mental, social, emotional, and spiritual dimensions. Within the United Nations (UN) system (https://www.un.org/en/global-issues/health) is the World Health Organization (WHO), whose role is to protect and promote health worldwide. The WHO defines health as "a state of complete physical, mental, and social well-being and not merely the absence of disease or infirmity" and as "one of the fundamental rights of every human being without distinction of race, religion, political belief, economic or social condition" (WHO, n.d.-a). The WHO further-more expands the definition of health to include the responsibility of governments to provide adequate health and social measures. The United States is a member state of the WHO.

Social Determinants of Health Influencing Older Adult Well-Being and Care

Since 1990, the U.S. Department of Health and Human Services (USDHHS), through the Healthy People initiatives, has identified national goals and objectives to achieve healthier lives across the lifespan of older adults. Within the span of each decade there are general leading health indicators, and population-specific indicators, where key objectives and improvements are measured and monitored over time. In addition, Healthy People 2030 addresses Social Determinants of Health (SDOH) that are inherently associated with the well-being of persons across their lifespan: "Social determinants of health (SDOH) are the conditions in the environments where people are born, live, learn, work, play, worship, and age that affect a wide range of health, functioning, and quality-of-life outcomes and risks" (USDHHS, n.d.-a).

The five domains in Social Determinants of Health are (1) economic stability, (2) education access and quality, (3) health care access and quality, (4) neighborhood and built environment, and (5) social and community context (see Figure 1.2). With reference to older adults, social determinants of health are keenly important. The World Health Organization (WHO) gives the following definition:

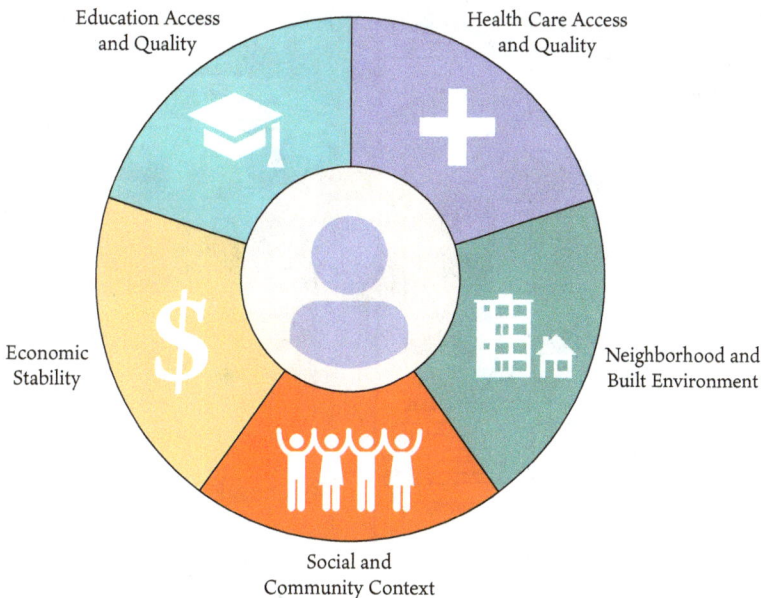

FIGURE 1.2   Social Determinants of Health

The social determinants of health (SDH) are the non-medical factors that influence health outcomes. They are the conditions in which people are born, grow, work, live, and age, and the wider set of forces and systems shaping the conditions of daily life. These forces and systems include economic policies and systems, development agendas, social norms, social policies and political systems. (WHO, n.d.-c)

Health Equity

Given the holistic definition of health and social determinants that influence health provided above, it is realistic to discuss health equity. Health equity refers to the *absence* of unfair differences in health that are social, economic, demographic, or geographic (WHO, n.d.-c). Figure 1.3 illustrates this point, in that equality does not necessarily mean equity.

Equity is social justice in health throughout the life cycle continuum (Braveman, 2014). In a sense, Healthy People 2030 provides testimony to the existence of health inequities among populations. Identified in Healthy People 2030 are explicit goals, actions, and metrics by which health care professionals, systems, and government agencies measure progress and effectiveness in achieving goals. The Healthy People 2030 initiatives are an approach to reducing disparities. The topic of health disparities is further discussed in Chapter 6.

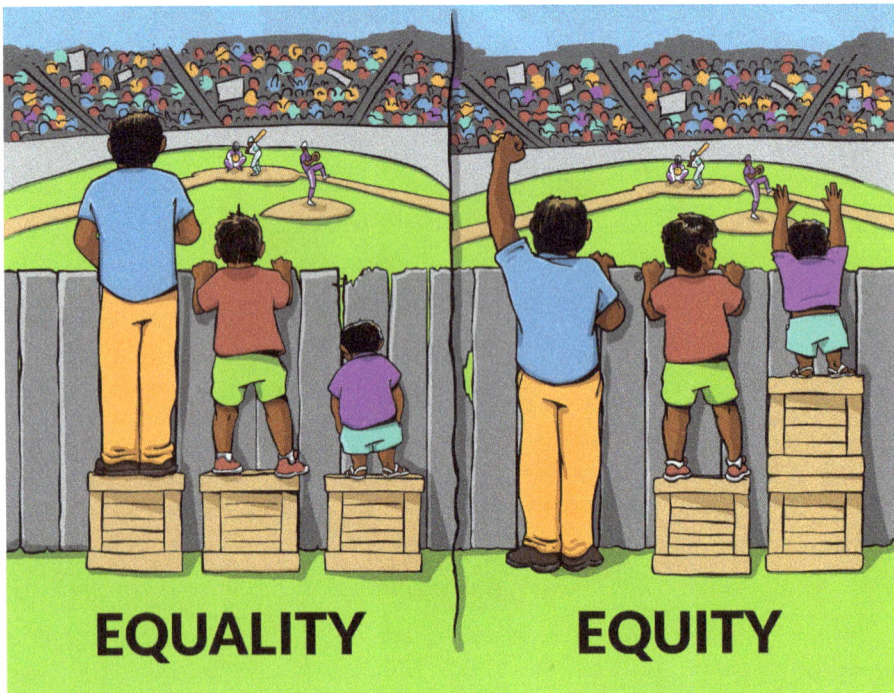

FIGURE 1.3 Health Equity

Case Study

Consider the following questions in this case study that brings to bear the previous discussion of social determinants of health, health equity, and the concept of praxis:

- What are the social determinants of health that may influence this older adult's health?

- Is health equity achieved for this older adult? Why or why not?

- What thoughts or reflections do you have about the community in which this older adult and her granddaughter live?

- If it were *you* as the nurse in this case study, what questions would you be asking of yourself as the health care professional involved in this community?

- If it were *you* as the nurse in this case study, what do you see as transformative actions that you would undertake as an individual, or in collaboration with others, that would make a difference?

Audra Marie Cohen-Brown is a 70-year-old widowed African American woman. She is soft-spoken and strong in her faith. She is known as a kind person in her circle of friends, always offering others a ride when in need and always bringing words of comfort and hope when others are ill, homebound, or feeling down. In the living room of her tiny duplex in the impoverished south part of town are pictures and small tapestries of Martin Luther King Jr., President John F. Kennedy, and framed quotations from scripture. Her duplex is well lit with natural sunlight, well kept, and has safe, clean running water, electricity, and a wall heater. There is no air-conditioning, but during the hot summer months, Audra keeps a large fan on to circulate the air. She regularly attends mass, weekly Bible studies, and choir practice at the Catholic Church near her home, when she is well. Her fellow parishioners are her closest friends and sole source of social support. In spite of her life hardships and stressors, Audra maintains her faith in God, who she believes is her wellspring of hope and a personal source of strength.

She is the sole guardian and custodian of a female minor, her 8-year-old granddaughter Lois, who she is raising alone. Audra is a role model for her granddaughter. She has enrolled her granddaughter in the Catholic school affiliated with her church. Lois is soft-spoken, well-mannered, bright, witty, and excels at her schoolwork. Lois's mother, a chronic substance abuser, lives 350 miles away in another part of the state and has had little or no communication with Audra or Lois.

Audra manages to care for herself and her granddaughter on her Social Security income and some savings. She is on Medi-Cal. She is functional, mobile, and able to perform activities of daily living and instrumental activities of daily living. She drives her car that she owns wherever she and her granddaughter need to go— church, school, grocery shopping, and Audra's doctor appointments. Audra wears eyeglasses, partial dentures, and has no other sensory impairments. She is 5 feet 3 inches tall, moderately obese, and is on prescribed medication for her hypertension. Granddaughter Lois is in good health, having an occasional cold during the winter months. Lois is slender but within normal height and weight for her age.

The neighborhood where Audra and her granddaughter live is unsafe for outdoor activity and recreation. This south part of town is frequented by gangs. There are no green spaces, playgrounds, walkways, or nature paths to enjoy. Unlike the north part of town, where there is visible evidence of greater wealth, there are no streetlights, and roads and sidewalks are in poor repair. It is common to see exterior windows of homes bound by vertical iron bars that are bolted down. The south part of town, according to city census data, has a population of 100,000. The median annual income of persons in the south is $54,000 in contrast to the $60,000 median annual income of the town overall.

Most of the socialization for Lois is with other children who attend church or with her classmates while school is in session. The nearest decent park is across town. The nearest grocery store is also across town, and Audra takes the freeway to get there. Audra's doctor is located in the north part of town and she makes the trek across the freeway to keep her appointments. For the residents of this community, many make the same trek across the freeway for needed supplies, groceries, and health care. Furthermore, many are migrant farm workers who have little time for health care visits nor the means to pay for them.

Through the advocacy of some active parishioners in Audra's church and the Sisters of the Immaculate Heart affiliated with the church, there is now a parish nurse, Eduardo, who makes home health visits to families in Audra's community. He is able to perform health assessments on persons of all ages, provides just-in-time health teaching, and generally seizes opportunities to help people lead healthier lives. He is able to make referrals to a social worker and other health care providers as needed. He administers seasonal flu shots and other immunizations after mass on Sundays. At the request of parishioners, Eduardo provided masks, hand gel, and COVID test kits to residents of this south community through collaboration with the public health department. Eduardo is concerned about other parishioners and community-dwelling older adults who are unable to travel or have no means of travel to get flu shots or personal protective equipment at church. The nurse is concerned about distances people must travel to access health care and grocery stores along with the lack of public transportation, a fire station, and other community amenities such as parks, playgrounds, and a public library. The nurse has established trust over time, and the members of this community want more parish nurses and ready, easy access to health care services.

As you, the learner, read through this case study, discuss the social determinants of health, health equity, and the nurse's role and professional practice in light of the code of ethics. More importantly, also consider praxis as defined by Freire (1970): "The action and reflection of people upon their world in order to transform it."

Chapter Summary

This chapter provides the learner with affirming assumptions relevant to older adults and core foundations essential to care of the older adult. Core values, the code of ethics, and praxis, or reflective practice, centers the nurse on responsibility to self, to others in their care, and the social context in which nursing care is given. Social determinants of health and health equity are factors innately connected with the health and well-being of older adults.

Glossary

Assumption: A statement held to be true, even though it may not be scientifically proven; it is a premise or a presupposition that forms the basis of reasoning, rationale, or from which conclusions may be drawn.

Code of ethics: A statement of beliefs, values, and principles that guide the practice and conduct of a profession or members of an association or organization. The American Nurses Association (ANA) Code of Ethics is reviewed and revised periodically to reflect dynamic changes in practice, the health care needs of society, and personal and professional growth.

Comportment: Dignified manner or conduct, essential to effective relationships, communication, and collaboration with patients, members of the health care team, and nurse colleagues.

Critical reflection: A deeply inward, honest, and systematic appraisal of one's thoughts, actions, and experiences for the purposes of acquiring insight, awareness, and effective change. Critical reflection may take place on a personal level or within a group or organization.

Health: A concept that describes or defines one's holistic being in multiple dimensions of physical, psycho-socio-emotional, spiritual, cultural, and environmental health across life stages, time, and geography. Definitions of health often include the person or patient, the environment, one's professional role and responsibility to persons or patients and to society, the context in which health occurs, and optimum states toward which to strive. Health may be defined on a personal, group, community, organizational, or national level. A widely accepted and brief definition of health is that of the World Health Organization (WHO, n.d.-c).

Health equity: Conditions in which persons have full opportunity to attain their full health potential and no one is disadvantaged by social position or circumstance. Conditions are those of health care access; health care infrastructure; and social, environmental, economic, cultural, and political determinants within communities.

Mission statement: A statement of values and purpose that governs one's choices, actions, and relationships. Mission statements are created at the personal, group, or organizational levels.

Older adult: Chronologically, an older adult is one who is 65+ years of age as defined by the National Institute on Aging. Centenarians are persons of 100–109 years, supercentenarians are those who live to be 110 years of age. In other areas of the world, an older adult is one between the ages of 50 to 65 years of age. Cultures vary in their definitions of older adult.

Praxis: An intentional and purposeful process of reflection and action creating an awareness of self, relationships, or conditions leading to positive change, growth, or transformation.

Social determinants: Conditions in environments where people are born, live, learn, work, play, worship, and age that affect health. Healthy People 2030 categorizes these conditions as economic stability, education access and quality, health care access and quality, neighborhood and built environment, and social and community context.

Social justice: Understanding societal inequalities that create oppression and disadvantage, and taking action toward social change.

References

American Nurses Association (ANA). (2015). *Code of ethics.* https://www.nursingworld.org/practice-policy/nursing-excellence/ethics/code-of-ethics-for-nurses/

American Nurses Association (ANA). (2019). *Gerontological nursing: Scope and standards of practice* (2nd ed.).

Braveman, P. (2014). What is health equity: And how does a life-course approach take us further toward it? *Maternal Child Health Journal, 18,* 366–72. https://doi.org/10.1007/s10995-013-1226-9.

Chinn, P. L., Kramer, M. K., & Sitzman, K. (2022). *Knowledge development in nursing: Theory and process* (11th ed.). Elsevier.

Clickner, D. A., & Shirey, M. R. (2013). Professional comportment: The missing element in nursing practice. *Nursing Forum, 18*(2), 106–13.

Fowler, M. D. M. (2015a). *Guide to the code of ethics for nurses with interpretive statements: Development, interpretation, and application* (2nd ed.). American Nurses Association.

Fowler, M. D. M. (2015b). *Guide to nursing's social policy statement: Understanding the profession from social contract to social covenant.* American Nurses Association.

Freire, P. (1970). *Pedagogy of the oppressed* (M. S. Ramos, Tr.). The Seabury Press.

Fry, M., MacGregor, C., Ruperto, K., Jarrett, K., Wheeler, J., Fong, J., & Fetchet, W. (2013). Nursing praxis, compassionate caring and interpersonal relations: An observational study. *Australasian Emergency Nursing Journal, 16,* 37–44. http://dx.doi.org/10.1016/j.aenj.2013.02.003.

Hills, M., Watson, J., & Chantal, C. (2021). *Creating a caring science curriculum: A relational emancipatory pedagogy for nursing* (2nd ed.). Springer.

Kagan, P. N., Smith, M. C., Cowling, R. W., III, & Chinn, P. L. (2009). A nursing manifesto: An emancipatory call for knowledge development, conscience, and praxis. *Nursing Philosophy, 11,* 67–84.

Keith, J. (1987). The right to health or the right to health care. *Nursing Praxis in New Zealand, 2*(3), 18–23.

Rafii, F., Nasrabadi, N., & Tehrani, F. J. (2022). Factors involved in praxis in nursing practice. A qualitative study. *Journal of Caring Sciences, 11*(2), 83–93. https://doi.org/10.34172/jcs.2021.020.

Rolfe, G. (2006). Nursing praxis and the science of the unique. *Nursing Science Quarterly, 19*(1), 39–43. https://doi.org/10.1177/0894318405284128.

United States Department of Health & Human Services (USDHHS). (n.d.-a). *Healthy people 2030.* Retrieved July 27, 2022, from https://health.gov/healthypeople/objectives-and-data/social-determinants-health

United States Department of Health & Human Services (USDHHS). (n.d.-b). *National standards for culturally and linguistically appropriate services (CLAS) in health and health care.* Retrieved July 27, 2022, from https://thinkculturalhealth.hhs.gov/clas

World Health Organization (WHO). (n.d.-a). Constitution. *Governance.* Retrieved July 11, 2022, from https://www.who.int/about/governance/constitution

World Health Organization (WHO). (n.d.-b). Health equity. *Social determinants of health.* Retrieved July 11, 2022, from https://www.who.int/health-topics/social-determinants-of-health#tab=tab_3

World Health Organization (WHO). (n.d.-c). Overview. *Social determinants of health.* Retrieved July 11, 2022, from https://www.who.int/health-topics/social-determinants-of-health#tab=tab_1

Selected Bibliography

Benner, P., Sutphen, M., Keonard-Kahn, V., & Day, L. (2008). Formation and everyday ethical comportment. *American Journal of Critical Care, 17,* 473–76.

Butterfield, P. G. (1990). Thinking upstream: Nurturing a conceptual understanding of the societal context of health behavior. *Advances in Nursing Science, 12*(2), 1–8.

Cowling, R., Chinn, P., Hagedorn, S. (n.d.). *Manifesto with markers for citation.* NurseManifest: A call to conscience and action. Retrieved July 1, 2023, from https://nursemanifest.com/a-nursing-manifesto-a-call-to-conscience-and-action/manifesto-with-markers-for-citation/

Holmes, C., & Warelow, P. (2000). Nursing as normative praxis. *Nursing Inquiry, 7,* 175–81.

Kemmis, S. (2023). Education for living well in a world worth living in. In K. E. Reimer, M. Kaukko, S. Windsor, K. Mahon, & S. Kemmis (Eds.), *Living well in a world worth living in for all, Vol. 1: Current practices of social justice, sustainability, and wellbeing* (pp. 13–25). Springer. https://doi.org/10.1007/978-981-19-7985-9_2

Rafii, F., Nasrabadi, A. N., & Tehrani, F. J. (2022). Factors involved in praxis in nursing practice: A qualitative study. *Journal of Caring Sciences, 11*(2), 83–93. https://doi.1034172/jcs.2021.020

Image Credits

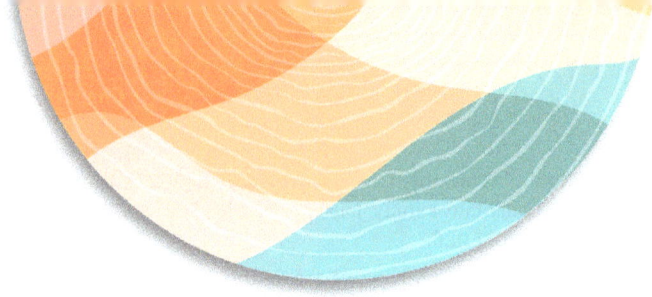

GLOBAL PHENOMENON OF AGING

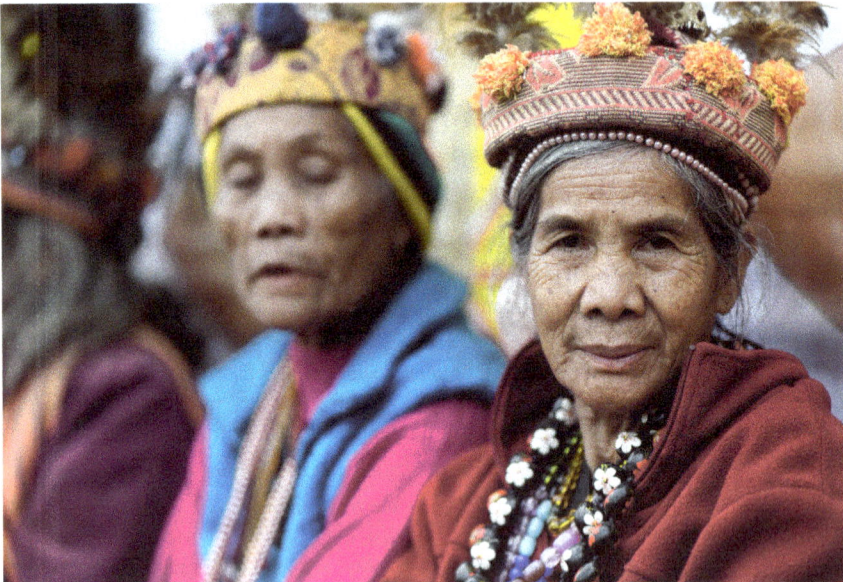

Image 2.1

Overview

This chapter explores broad aging trends. Knowledge development and scientific advances have led to care and treatment interventions that facilitate health in advanced age. An understanding of aging demographics, trends, and factors influencing health in advanced age are foundational in promoting health.

Outcomes

The learner:

1. Describes current global aging population shifts

2. Describes factors that contribute to an increase in aging populations

3. Discusses the impact/implications of care of older aging populations in developed and underdeveloped economies

4. Compares and contrasts the Sustainable Development Goals (SDGs) and Healthy People 2030 Objectives as they relate to aging populations

Aging Defined

Normal physiological changes occur with aging, and these are well documented in the scientific literature. *Aging* as defined by the World Health Organization (WHO) is explained in biological terms. It is molecular and cellular death that ultimately results in decreased capacity and higher risk of disease (WHO, 2022). At the cellular level, there is evidence that biochemical changes in aging occur. Beyond the cellular level are body organ systems, working interdependently to carry out metabolic functions. There is also evidence that human-environment interactions may result in changes that affect cellular and organ function, which may lead to vulnerability in the older adult. For example, exposure to smog, cigarette smoke, radiation, and pesticides can lead to cellular damage. Aging is influenced by other factors such as transitions and major life events.

The United Nations (UN) definition of aging populations are persons 65 years of age and older. The UN takes a much broader view and advocates for the recognition of aging, contributions of older adults to society, human rights, and the responsibility of nations in protecting those rights (United Nations, 2022; United Nations, 1991).

Another dimension of aging is the context in which aging occurs. This is the context, comprising culture and the perceived values and attitudes toward aging and older adults. Family may readily transmit or communicate values and attitudes toward aging. The context in which aging occurs is the sociocultural community context where persons, families, and groups live, work, and play. The sociocultural community is a broader reflection of values and attitudes toward aging and older adults as expressed through infrastructure and safe environments—ready access to nutritious food, health care, recreational spaces, housing, public transportation, and programs. While older adults may experience varied life transitions that affect them differently, the extent to which older adults live healthy, active, and independent lives is in part fostered by community infrastructure—the built environment and social programs. At a much broader level are local, county, and state governments, who support and finance community infrastructure and programs, and develop policies to meet population needs.

Where in the World Are People Aging?

Concentrations of aging populations are found in every world region. In 2020, persons age 60 and older outnumbered children 5 years of age or younger. By 2030, 1 out of 6 persons will be 60 years of age or older, and this population and will number 1.4 billion persons worldwide. The World Health Organization notes that between 2015 and 2050, persons 60 years of age and older will nearly double, from 12% to 22% of the world's population. By 2050 persons 80 years of age and older will triple, resulting in 426 million persons by 2050 (WHO, n.d.-c, n.d.-d).

Europe

Regionally, Europe has the oldest population, with adults age 65 or older comprising 19% of the total population, or in other words, 1 in 5 persons are age 65 or older. International migration will be an influencing factor related to population size (PRB, 2022a).

Americas

The region also has the world's oldest population, with adults ages 65 and older accounting for almost 1 in 5 (19%) of the total population. Future population size will likely be determined mainly by international migration (PRB, 2022c).

Africa

Africa includes the areas of Northern Africa and the sub-Saharan Africa subregions of Eastern Africa, Middle Africa, Southern Africa, and Western Africa. The population is projected to grow from 1.4 billion in 2022 to 2.5 billion in 2050 (60% of the projected global population growth during this period). However, as fertility declines from high to low levels, so will the young dependent population relative to those within working ages. This may provide an opportunity for economic growth (PRB, 2022b).

Asia

The share of adults age 65 and older also varies within Asia, ranging from 5% in Central Asia to 15% in East Asia (PRB, 2022d).

Oceania

This region is home to some of the world's youngest areas and some of its oldest. In Samoa, Solomon Islands, Nauru, and Vanuatu, nearly 40% of people are under age 15. In Australia and New Zealand, 18% and 19% of the population is under age 15, respectively, and 17% are ages 65 and older (PRB 2022e).

United States

The United States mirrors the global aging trend. In 2023, persons age 60 or older number at 82,862,258 and comprise 24.4% of the U.S. population. By 2030, this population is projected to increase to 92,702,683. By 2050, population projections for this age demographic estimate 108,338,610 persons. These projections represent 26.1% and 27.9% of the total U.S. populations. By all projected estimates, the proportion of females is greater than that of males (WHO, n.d.-a); Table 2.1).

TABLE 2.1 United States Population of Adults Age 60+ Years

2023		Total Population	% of Population	Male Population	% of Males	Female Population	% of Females	Sex Ratio
		339,665,118	100.0	167,444,610	100.0	172,220,508	100.0	0.97
Age Group (Years of Age)	60+	8,286,258	24.4	37,842,232	22.6	45,020,026	26.1	0.84

2030		Total Population	% of Population	Male Population	% of Males	Female Population	% of Females	Sex Ratio
		355,100,730	100.0	175,173,907	100.0	179,926,823	100.0	0.97
Age Group (Years of Age)	60+	92,702,683	26.1	42,399,313	24.2	50,303,370	28.0	0.84

2050		Total Population	% of Population	Male Population	% of Males	Female Population	% of Females	Sex Ratio
		388,922,201	100.0	192,576,740	100.0	196,345,461	100.0	0.98
Age Group (Years of Age)	60*	108,338,610	27.9	49,950,939	25.9	58,387,671	29.7	0.86

Source: World Health Organization (n.d.-b). Ageing-demographics. Data portal: Number of persons aged 60 years or over (thousands). World Health Organization. https://platform.who.int/data/maternal-newborn-child-adolescent-ageing/ageing-data/ageing---demographics

In 2023, groups 80 years of age or greater made up 4.2% of the U.S. population. This older age group is also projected to comprise an increased percentage of the older adult population. It is expected that persons in this specific age group will account for 5.5% and 8.1% of the U.S. population in 2030 and 2050, respectively (Table 2.2).

TABLE 2.2 United States Population of Adults Age 80+ Years

2023							
Age Group (Years of Age)	Total Population	% of Population	Male Population	% of Males	Female Population	% of Females	Sex Ratio
	339,665,118	100.0	167,444,610	100.0	172,220,508	100.0	0.97
80–84	7,489,487	2.2	3,203,811	1.9	4,285,676	2.5	0.75
85–89	4,203,769	1.2	1,659,509	1.0	2,544,260	1.5	0.65
90–94	2,059,891	0.6	718,375	0.4	1,341,516	0.8	0.54
95–99	701,020	0.2	207,201	0.1	493,819	0.3	0.42
100+	108,974	0.0	26,973	0.0	82,001	0.0	0.33
2030							
Age Group (Years of Age)	Total Population	% of Population	Male Population	% of Males	Female Population	% of Females	Sex Ratio
	355,100,730	100.0	175,173,907	100.0	179,926,823	100.0	0.97
80–84	10,609,439	3.0	4,586,976	2.6	6,022,463	3.3	0.76
85–89	5,695,205	1.6	2,288,764	1.3	3,406,441	1.5	0.67
90–94	2,455,026	0.7	889,542	0.5	1,565,484	0.9	0.57
95–99	784,075	0.2	247,234	0.1	536,841	0.3	0.46
100+	139,533	0.0	37,653	0.0	101,900	0.1	0.37
2050							
Age Group (Years of Age)	Total Population	% of Population	Male Population	% of Males	Female Population	% of Females	Sex Ratio
	388,922,201	100.0	192,576,740	100.0	196,345,461	100.0	0.98
80–84	13,317,481	3.4	5,917,717	3.1	7,399,764	3.8	0.80
85–89	10,252,103	2.6	4,250,785	2.2	6,001,318	3.1	0.71
90–94	5,817,259	1.5	2,191,785	1.1	3,625,474	1.8	0.60
95–99	2,106,163	0.5	693,916	0.4	1,412,247	0.7	0.49
100+	385,732	0.1	109,644	0.1	276,088	0.1	0.40

Note: Extracted from United States Census Bureau, International Database (IDP), Population Estimates and Projections for 227 Countries and Areas, Population by Age, Older Five Year Age Groups (U.S. Census Bureau, 2023b)

In the U.S. in 2020, 51% of persons age 65 and older lived in nine states (ACL, 2022), California (6.0 million), Florida (4.6 million), and Texas (3.9 million), New York (3.4 million), Pennsylvania (2.4 million), Ohio (2.1 million), Illinois (2.1 million), North Carolina (1.8 million), and Michigan (1.8 million). In all states, including Washington, D.C., persons 65+ ranged from 6.1% to 21.2% of the respective population. In addition, 6.2% to 13.5% of 65+ lived below poverty. In Puerto Rico, persons 65+ make up 21.28% of the labor force (working or seeking work (ACL, 2022; U.S. Census Bureau, 2023a).

Significant growth is expected in the percentage of African Americans (13%), American Indians and Alaska Natives (0.7%), Asian Americans (8%), and Hispanic Americans (21%) who will be age 65 years and older by 2060 (Table 2.3).

TABLE 2.3 Demographic Characteristics of African Americans, American Indians and Alaska Natives, Asian Americans, Hispanic Americans, and Projected Growth Age 65 and Older

	Education (% with bachelor's degree or higher)	Grandparents (% responsible for basic needs of grandchildren ≤ age 18 living with them)	Median Income		Employment (% working or actively seeking work)		Projected Growth	
			Men	Women	Men	Women	2050	2060
African Americans	22%	35%	$25,106	$18,214	20.7%	16.4%	10,096,668	12,144,011
American Indians & Alaska Natives	21%	45%	18.7% at poverty rate	—	—	—	550,023	648,555
Asian Americans	43%	12%	$30,788	$21,815	25.6%	16.1%	6,353,765	7,858,517
Hispanic Americans	18%	19%	$21,357	$14,701	—	—	15,925,533	19,889,318

Sources: 2020 Profile of African Americans age 65 and older (ACL, 2021a). https://acl.gov/sites/default/files/Profile%20of%20OA/AAProfileReport2021.pdf
2020 Profile of American Indians and Alaska Natives age 65 and older (ACL, 2021b). https://acl.gov/sites/default/files/Profile%20of%20OA/AIANProfileReport2021.pdf
2020 Profile of Asian Americans age 65 and older (ACL, 2021c). https://acl.gov/sites/default/files/Profile%20of%20OA/AsianProfileReport2021.pdf
2020 Profile of Hispanic Americans age 65 and older (ACL, 2021d). https://acl.gov/sites/default/files/Profile%20of%20OA/HispanicProfileReport2021.pdf

Numbers of Older Adults by Country Rank

The countries with the largest numbers of older adults by rank from 1 to 5 are China, India, the United States, Japan, and the Russian Federation (Table 2.4). By percentage, Japan ranks first as the country with the largest percentage of older adults 65 years and older (28.2%). There are 35.58 million people who comprise 65+ age groups of 65–74, 75–84, and 85+ years of age. Within the age subgroups, 50% are age 65–74, 34% are age 75–84, and 16% are age 86 and older (Table 2.5).

TABLE 2.4 Countries with the Largest Number of Older Adults

Rank	Country	# 65+ (in millions)	% 65+ (of total population)	# Total Population (in millions)
1	China	166.37	11.9	1398.03
2	India	84.9	6.1	1391.89
3	United States	52.76	16	329.15
4	Japan	35.58	28.2	126.8
5	Russian Federation	21.42	14.6	146.73
6	Brazil	17.79	8.5	209.33
7	Germany	17.78	21.4	83.1
8	Indonesia	15.16	5.6	268.42
9	Italy	13.76	22.8	60.34
10	France	13.16	20.3	64.83
11	United Kingdom	12.24	18.3	66.83
12	Pakistan	9.31	4.3	216.57
13	Mexico	9.17	7.2	126.58
14	Spain	8.99	19.1	47.07
15	Bangladesh	8.35	5.1	163.67
16	South Korea	7.83	15.1	51.85
17	Thailand	7.61	11.5	66.37
18	Turkey	7.27	8.8	82.61
19	Ukraine	6.94	16.5	42.04
20	Poland	6.72	17.5	38.4

Sources: Countries with the oldest populations in the world: Top 50 countries with the largest percentage of older adults (PRB, 2020). https://www.prb.org/resources/countries-with-the-oldest-populations-in-the-world/
United Nations Population Division, World Population Prospects 2019. https://population.un.org/wpp/Download/Standard/Population/
Toshiko Kaneda, Charlotte Greenbaum, and Kaitlyn Patierno, 2019 World Population Data Sheet (Washington, DC: Population Reference Bureau, 2019).

In comparison, the United States ranks number 36 among the top 50 countries with the largest percentage of older adults age 65+ (16%). Twenty-nine percent (29%) of older adults age 65+ account for the 75–84 age group, and 13% are age 85 and over (Table 2.5).

TABLE 2.5 Countries with the Largest Percentage of Older Adults

Rank	Country	% 65+*	Age 65–74	Age 75–84	Age 85 and over	65+Population (in millions)	Total (in millions)
1	Japan	28.2	50	34	16	35.58	126.18
2	Italy	22.8	49	35	16	13.76	60.34
3	Finland	21.9	58	30	12	1.21	5.52
4	Portugal	21.8	51	35	14	2.24	10.27
5	Greece	21.8	48	35	17	2.33	10.70
6	Germany	21.4	47	39	14	17.78	83.1
7	Bulgaria	21.3	59	31	9	1.49	6.98
8	Croatia	20.4	54	34	12	0.83	4.05
9	France	20.3	54	29	17	13.16	64.83
10	Latvia	20.3	50	36	15	0.39	1.91
11	Serbia	20.2	--	--	--	1.40	6.94
12	Sweden	19.9	54	33	13	2.05	10.29
13	Lithuania	19.8	49	36	15	0.55	2.79
14	Estonia	19.8	50	36	13	0.26	1.33
15	Denmark	19.6	58	31	11	1.14	5.82
16	Czechia	19.6	61	29	10	2.09	10.67
17	Slovenia	19.6	54	33	13	0.41	2.09
18	Hungary	19.3	59	31	10	1.89	9.77
19	Malta	19.2	60	30	10	0.10	0.50
20	Spain	19.1	49	33	18	8.99	47.07
24	United Kingdom	18.3	54	32	14	12.24	66.83
31	Canada	17.2	58	29	13	6.44	37.41
33	Hong Kong, China	16.4	58	27	15	1.23	7.52
36	United States	16	58	29	13	52.76	329.15
44	Russian Federation	14.6	59	31	10	21.42	146.73

Sources: Countries with the oldest populations in the world: Top 50 countries with the largest percentage of older adults (PRB, 2020). https://www.prb.org/resources/countries-with-the-oldest-populations-in-the-world/ United Nations Population Division, World Population Prospects 2019, https://population.un.org/wpp/Download/ Standard/Population/, and Toshiko Kaneda, Charlotte Greenbaum, and Kaitlyn Patierno, 2019 World Population Data Sheet (Washington, DC: Population Reference Bureau, 2019).

---

* Breakdown of 65+ population (totaling 100%) across three columns showing age ranges of 65–74, 75–84, and 85+

The Pandemic and Aging Populations

One must acknowledge the impact of COVID-19 upon aging populations and global demographics. From January 2020 to December 2021, 14.9 million excess deaths were due to the COVID pandemic (Table 2.6). Older persons in households overall have been much more susceptible to COVID, with a higher mortality rate than younger age groups. Frailty, comorbidities in older adults, and country control and mitigation of the epidemic are key factors associated with COVID deaths in the elderly (United Nations, 2020). Overall, excess deaths in the U.S. due to COVID as a percent of total deaths in 2020–2021 was between 10% and 14%, with older adults at the highest risk of death from COVID. Other countries fared less (5%–9%), or greater, with 15% or more of total deaths in Western, Central, and South Asia, and more than 20% in Eastern Europe, Central and South America attributable to COVID (Population Reference Bureau, 2022f).

TABLE 2.6 Excess Pandemic Deaths as Percentage of Total Deaths January 2020–December 2021

	Population (millions) Mid-2022	Percent of Population Age 65+	Excess Deaths Due to COVID-19 Pandemic, 2020–2021 Annual Average			Population Fully Vaccinated Against COVID-19 (%)*
			No. of Excess Deaths	Excess Deaths per 100,000 population	Excess Deaths as % of Total Deaths	
World	7,963	10	7,455,097	96	12	62
More Developed	1,270	20	1,824,632	142	11	70
Less Developed	6,694	8	5,721,468	87	11	60
Least Developed	1,126	4	503,787	47	7	--
High Income	1,241	19	1,127,703	90	9	74
Middle Income	5,953	9	5,985,461	102	13	64
Upper Middle Income	2,527	13	2,053,784	82	10	77
Lower Middle Income	3,427	6	3,91,678	118	15	54
Low Income	738	3	330,795	47	7	17

Source: World population data sheet 2022: Special focus on the demographic impacts of Covid 19 (PRB, 2022f). https://2022-wpds.prb.org/special_focus/special-focus-on-covid-19/#mortality

---

*   John Hopkins Coronavirus Resource Center

Country Economies

Economic metrics reflect the ability and capacity of communities to provide programs and necessary infrastructure that facilitate healthy aging, health promotion, and disease prevention. By 2050, it is expected that 80% of older persons will be living in lower-middle-income countries (WHO, 2022, n.d.-f; Table 2.7).

TABLE 2.7 Income Group: Older Adult Age 60+ Years (Thousands) for All WHO Regions: Africa, Americas, Eastern Mediterranean, Europe, Global, South-East Asia, Western Pacific

Year	2023 (All)	2023	2030 (All)	2030	2050 (All)	2050
Global	1,144,157		1,416,984		2,132,389	
		Males/ Females		Males/ Females		Males/ Females
Low Income (GNI* $1,085)	37,541	16,684/ 20,858	48,869	21,881/ 26,988	101,970	46,486/ 55,484
Lower Middle Income (GNI $1,086–$4,255)	333,247	155,249/ 177,997	423,771	197,805/ 225,965	760,956	355,152/ 405,804
Upper Middle Income (GNI $4,256–$13,205)	445,345	199,313/ 246,032	573,987	258,767/ 315,221	823,263	379,827/ 443,346
High Income (GNI $13,206 or <)	324,154	147,563/ 176,591	365,514	168,290/ 197,224	438,996	206,883/ 232,114

Sources:
World development indicators: The world by income and region (World Bank, 2021). https://datatopics.worldbank.org/world-development-indicators/the-world-by-income-and-region.html
Gross National Income (GNI) per capita, Atlas method (current US$): World bank national accounts data, and Organisation for Economic Co-operation and Development (OECD) national accounts data files (World Bank, 2023b). https://data.worldbank.org/indicator/NY.GNP.PCAP.CD
WHO MNCAH data portal: World bank income group: Global, high income, low income, lower middle income, upper middle income (WHO, n.d.-f). https://platform.who.int/data/maternal-newborn-child-adolescent-ageing

---

* GNI; Gross national income per capita in US dollars; a strong indicator of the standard of living of an average citizen in the country, the gross domestic product, plus net receipts from abroad of compensation of employees, property income, and net taxes less subsidies on production.

The World Bank classifies income economies of countries utilizing the Gross National Income (GNI) per capita. The GNI is the dollar value of a country's final yearly income divided by its population. A detailed methodology, the Atlas method, is used to calculate GNI. For the current 2023 fiscal year, high-income economies are those with a GNI per capita (in US dollars) of $13,206 or more; upper-middle-income economies are those with a GNI per capita between $4,256 and $13,205; lower-middle-income economies are those with a GNI per capita between $1,086 and $4,255; low-income economies are defined as those with a GNI per capita of $1,085 or less in 2021 (World Bank, 2023a). The reader may access the classification of income economies by World Health Organization (WHO) regions, and by country, through this World Bank data.

Living Arrangements

Older adults have varied living arrangements. Living arrangements are important, as they are a determinant of well-being. In addition, this topic has societal implications as it affects community infrastructure, support systems, services, socioeconomics, and the overall well-being of older adults. Living arrangements of older adults and their relationship to household members are described as (a) living independently, (b) living with children under or older than 20 years of age, (c) living with extended family, (d) skip-generation households, and (e) non-relative households (United Nations, 2020; see glossary). These descriptions exclude those living in institutions.

Developed countries have a greater proportion of older adults who live alone. Their health status and having sufficient resources allow them to live independently. They may rely on adult children who live independently, siblings, other relatives, and friends for social support and contact. The proportion of older adults living alone in less developed countries varies. Older adults living alone are more vulnerable, with greater reliance on children and kin for support. There is a greater proportion of older women living alone than men, and they are more likely to be living in poverty.

There is a greater proportion of intergenerational households in urban areas in developing countries. Economic downturns, housing shortages, employment prospects for adult children, and familial and cultural traditions contribute to intergenerational households. Older men are more likely to live with children under age 20, whereas older women are more likely to live with children older than age 20.

Skip-Generation Households

Extended family households that include relatives such as grandchildren, nieces, or nephews afford older adults emotional and practical support. A type of extended family household that has become increasingly prevalent is the skip-generation household, consisting of grandparents and grandchildren. Essentially, members of the immediate generation (i.e., parents) are absent. Factors giving rise to skip-generation households are parental loss of custody, incarceration, substance abuse, and death. The HIV/AIDS epidemic and consequent mortality, international migration for economic reasons, and armed conflict are other important factors that have given rise to skip-generation households. For some world regions data are not available or not reported, or data is less than 1.0%. (United Nations, 2020; see Table 2.8).

TABLE 2.8 Living Arrangements Among Persons Aged 65 Years or Older, by Gender, 2006–2015

World Region/ Country	Percentage of persons age 65 years or older who are:							
	Living alone		Living with spouse only		Living with children		Living with grandchildren	
	Women	Men	Women	Men	Women	Men	Women	Men
	24.0	11.0	23.0	24.0	--	--	--	--
Sub-Saharan Africa	13	7.9	5.8	13.7	--	--	--	--
Northern Africa and Western Asia	--	--	--	--	--	--	--	--
Central and Southern Asia	7.9	2.4	8.7	18.4	--	--	--	--
Eastern and Southeastern Asia	--	--	--	--	--	--	--	--
Latin America and the Caribbean	16.9	11.9	16.2	27.6	--	--	--	--
Oceania excluding Australia and New Zealand	--	--	--	--	--	--	--	--
Australia and New Zealand	33.5	18.1	44.0	59.9	--	--	--	--
Europe and Northern America	36.8	17.7	32.8	56.0	--	--	--	--
Africa								
Eastern Africa								

continued

TABLE 2.8 *continued*

Burundi	20.5	5.0	5.3	13.7	14.3	36.8	32.0	15.6
Madagascar	11.0	7.1	6.6	10.4	5.0	16.4	28.4	18.6
Rwanda	18.1	7.5	5.2	11.9	12.6	30.4	28.8	15.4
Uganda	11.7	11.1	2.3	7.3	5.3	15.2	30.0	16.7
Zambia	11.0	6.6	5.7	12.3	7.7	19.6	24.0	16.4
Middle Africa								
Democratic Republic of the Congo	16.4	6.0	5.0	16.0	3.6	16.3	25.0	16.9

Source:United Nations. (2020). World population ageing 2020 highlights: Living arrangements of older persons. www.un.org/development/desa/pd

Skip-generation households in low- and middle-income countries are often economically disadvantaged, with poorer health outcomes and increasing physical, emotional, and mental strain on grandparents who are raising active young children (Zimmer & Treleaven, 2020). In spite of these challenges, research evidence supports benefits and positive aspects of grandparents' having primary responsibility for grandchildren. Maintaining harmony of life is a phenomenon embracing positivity, life perspective, courage, hope, and intrinsic motivation (Komjakraphan & Chansawang, 2015). Zimmer and Treleaven (2020) point out that grandparents benefit psychologically by having a sense of purpose, better mental health, and slower health decline. Families who are left behind often fare better economically from remittances sent home to them by migrating parents working abroad. Children of migrating parents in skip-generation households also have less food insecurity and lower rates of malnutrition. In addition, they are more likely to stay in school.

Contributing Factors to the Growth of Older Adult Populations

The global trend of a growing aging population can be attributed to multiple factors. Public health promotion and health messages are widely disseminated to general and targeted populations. Information is available and accessible through the internet, news outlets, and social media campaigns. Information and media are also broadcast in different languages and formats that have broad appeal. Visual images, including product labels and infographics, are examples of ways in which public health promotion and health messages are communicated. Lifestyle choices, such as physical activity, nutrition, sleep, and rest, have an impact on health and longevity, and these are already well documented in the literature.

Advances in scientific knowledge and technology have led to care and treatment interventions that facilitate health in advanced age. Health examinations and preventive screening are essential in health maintenance and illness prevention. Evidence-based screening tools can be used to assess and evaluate health and well-being (Hartford Institute for Geriatric Nursing, n.d.). Public health information has raised greater awareness of screening for age-related changes such as vision and hearing. Public awareness of colorectal and breast cancer screening along with chronic illness prevention (hypertension, heart and lung disease, diabetes, osteoporosis) may prevent severe disability in later years.

The U.S. Department of Health and Human Services uses an evidence-driven approach to identifying national objectives to be achieved across the life cycle over the next decade (USDHHS, n.d.-a). Leading health indicators (LHIs) in the older adult population are high-priority indicators that impact major causes of death and disease in the U.S. These indicators are an important focus for community resources and efforts to improve health and well-being of older adults.

Social Determinants of Health

Other significant factors, which may vary by region and for groups and individuals, contribute to overall health in advanced age. Social determinants of health (SDOH; USDHHS, n.d.-b) consist of five domains that influence health, functioning, quality of life, outcomes, and risks. The goals of the Healthy People 2030 initiative are to improve in each of the five domains (see Figure 1.2, Chapter 1):

- Economic stability: Help people earn steady incomes that allow them to meet their health needs.

- Education access and quality: Increase educational opportunities and help children and adolescents do well in school.

- Health care access and quality: Increase access to comprehensive, high-quality health care services.

- Neighborhood and built environment: Create neighborhood environments that provide health and safety.

- Social and community context: Increase social and community support.

While education access and quality are defined specifically for children and adolescents, older adults may also benefit from education access through various programs as lifelong learners. Such access (e.g., high school completion, degree completion, continuing education programs) may improve quality of life in advanced age.

Evidence-based resources, screening tools, and monitoring and progress toward goal achievement in each domain of SDOH are readily accessible. Social determinants of health have profound influences on health care outcomes, namely in health care access and quality. The latter topic will be explored more fully in Chapter 5.

Research literature provides evidence of linkages between social determinants of health and health outcomes (Battle & Clarke, 2022; Fastame, Ruiu, & Mulas, 2021; Hosseinpoor, Williams, Itani, & Chatterji, 2012; Poulain, Poulain, Herm, Errigo, Chrysohoou, Legrand, Passarino, Stazi, Voutekatis, Gonos, Francheschi, & Pes, 2021; Rapp, Ronchetti, & Sicsic, 2022).

Sustainable Development Goals (SDGs)

The UN has identified 17 Sustainable Development Goals (SDGs), comprehensive in scope and applicable to regions and communities worldwide (Figure 2.1). The SDGs affect persons across the life cycle. The 17 goals, developed by member states, recognize and acknowledge that ending deprivations requires health care strategies that improve health, address education inequalities, and promote economic growth. The goals also attend to climate change and preservation of natural resources, all of which impact health. Actions implemented to date and markers of achievement and progress are documented annually. Clearly evident in SDOH and SDGs are cross-cutting issues affecting all regions, populations, communities, groups, and individuals.

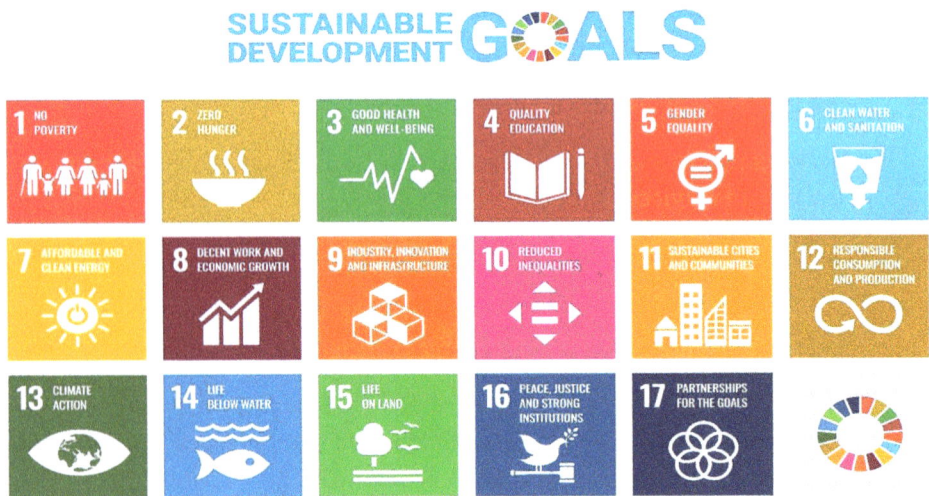

FIGURE 2.1   The UN's Sustainable Development Goals

An age-friendly world necessitates global effort and collaboration. Toward this end, the Madrid International Plan of Action on Aging and its accompanying legal instrument, Principles for Older Persons, was ratified by member states in 2002. Review and appraisal of both instruments occurred in February 2023 and continue in founding treatises for economic and social development of governments (United Nations, 1991, 2022).

Chapter Summary

This chapter provided an overview of current statistics and projected growth of the aging population in the U.S. and worldwide. Scientific knowledge, technological advancements, public health promotion, and preventive health screening in the field of aging have contributed to longevity. Research evidence points to the Social Determinants of Health as a vital aspect of overall health and well-being in advanced age. Healthy aging in societies must also consider social and economic development and the responsibilities of health care professionals, organizations, and governments in safeguarding the rights of older persons. The Sustainable Development Goals are a global call to action.

Glossary

Extended family households: Include one or more members from outside the nuclear family unit and no members who are not related to each other.

Living with children: Couple (married or unmarried) or single parent living with their children only (biological, adopted, foster children, stepchildren, and children-in-law, irrespective of ages).

Living with children under 20 years of age: The oldest coresident child is 0–19 years old.

Living with children 20 years of age or over: The oldest coresident child is age 20 years or older.

Living independently: An older person living alone or with a spouse or partner only.

Skip-generation households: Households consisting of grandparents and their grandchildren, with no one from the intermediate generation (parents of the grandchildren or children of the grandparents).

Source: World population ageing 2020 highlights: Living arrangements of older persons (United Nations, 2020). www.un/org/development/desa/pd/.

References

Administration for Community Living (ACL). (2021, May). *2020 profile of older Americans*. U.S. Department of Health and Human Services. https://acl.gov/sites/default/files/Profile%20 of%20OA/2020ProfileOlderAmericans_RevisedFinal.pdf

Administration for Community Living (ACL). (2021a). *2020 profile of African Americans age 65 and older*. U.S. Department of Health and Human Services. https://acl.gov/sites/default/files/ Profile%20of%20OA/AAProfileReport2021.pdf

Administration for Community Living (ACL). (2021b). *2020 profile of American Indians and Alaska Natives age 65 and older*. U.S. Department of Health and Human Services. https://acl. gov/sites/default/files/Profile%20of%20OA/AIANProfileReport2021.pdf

Administration for Community Living (ACL). (2021c). *2020 profile of Asian Americans age 65 and older*. U.S. Department of Health and Human Services. https://acl.gov/sites/default/files/Profile %20of%20OA/AsianProfileReport2021.pdf

Administration for Community Living (ACL). (2021d). *2020 profile of Hispanic Americans age 65 and older*. U.S. Department of Health and Human Services. https://acl.gov/sites/default/files/ Profile%20of%20OA/HispanicProfileReport2021.pdf

Administration for Community Living (ACL). (2022, November). *2021 profile of older Americans*. U.S. Department of Health and Human Services. https://acl.gov/sites/default/files/Profile%20 of%20OA/2021%20Profile%20of%20OA/2021ProfileOlderAmericans_508.pdf

Hartford Institute for Geriatric Nursing. (n.d.). *Try This:® Series*. https://hign.org/

Komjakraphan, P., & Chansawang, W. (2015). Maintaining harmony of life in skipped-generation households of the older adults. *Asian/Pacific Island Nursing Journal*, 1–7. https://doi.org/10.1177/ 2373665815569505

Population Reference Bureau (PRB). (2020). *Countries with the oldest populations in the world: Top 50 countries with the largest number of older adults*. https://www.prb.org/resources/countries-with-the-oldest-populations-in-the-world/

Population Reference Bureau (PRB). (2022a). *World population data sheet: Europe overview*. Retrieved February 23, 2023, from https://2022-wpds.prb.org/europe/

Population Reference Bureau (PRB). (2022b). *World population data sheet: Africa overview*. Retrieved February 23, 2023, https://2022-wpds.prb.org/africa/

Population Reference Bureau (PRB). (2022c). *World population data sheet: Americas overview*. Retrieved February 23, 2023, https://2022-wpds.prb.org/americas/

Population Reference Bureau (PRB). (2022d). *World population data sheet: Asia overview*. Retrieved February 23, 2023, https://2022-wpds.prb.org/asia/

Population Reference Bureau (PRB). (2022e). *World population data sheet: Oceania overview*. Retrieved February 23, 2023, https://2022-wpds.prb.org/oceania/

Population Reference Bureau (PRB). (2022f). *World population data sheet 2022: Special focus on the demographic impacts of Covid 19*. https://2022-wpds.prb.org/special_focus/special-focus-on-covid-19/#mortality

United Nations Population Division (2019). *World population prospects 2019*. https://population. un.org/wpp/Download/Standard/Population/

United Nations. (n.d.). *The 17 goals*. Department of Economic and Social Affairs, Sustainable Development. https://sdgs.un.org/goals

United Nations. (1991). *Universal instrument: United Nations principles for older persons, General Assembly resolution 46/91, adopted December 16, 1991*. https://www.ohchr.org/en/ instruments-mechanisms/instruments/united-nations-principles-older-persons

United Nations. (2020). *World population ageing 2020 highlights: Living arrangements of older persons.* www.un/org/development/desa/pd/

United Nations. (2022). *Fourth review and appraisal of the Madrid International Plan of Action on Ageing, 2002: Report of the Secretary General, Economic and Social Council, Commission for Social Development, 61st session, February 6–15, 2023,* https://documents-dds-ny.un.org/doc/UNDOC/GEN/N22/705/05/PDF/N2270505.pdf?OpenElement

United States Census Bureau. (2023a). *International database (IDB): Population estimates and projections for 227 countries and areas. Older age groups.* https://www.census.gov/data-tools/demo/idb/#/pop?COUNTRY_YEAR=2023&COUNTRY_YR_ANIM=2023&ANIM_PARAMS=2010,2060,1&menu=popViz&popPages=BYAGE&POP_YEARS=2023&FIPS_SINGLE=US&FIPS=US&ageGroup=O

United States Census Bureau. (2023b). *International database (IDB): Population estimates and projections for 227 countries and areas. Older five year age groups.* https://www.census.gov/data-tools/demo/idb/#/pop?COUNTRY_YEAR=2023&COUNTRY_YR_ANIM=2023&ANIM_PARAMS=2010,2060,1&menu=popViz&popPages=BYAGE&POP_YEARS=2023&FIPS_SINGLE=US&FIPS=US&ageGroup=O5

United States Department of Health and Human Services (USDHHS). (n.d.-a). *Healthy people 2030.* Office of Disease Prevention and Health Promotion. https://health.gov/healthypeople

United States Department of Health and Human Services (USDHHS). (n.d.-b). *Social determinants of health.* Office of Disease Prevention and Health Promotion. https://health.gov/healthypeople/priority-areas/social-determinants-health

World Bank. (2021). *World development indicators: The world by income and region.* https://datatopics.worldbank.org/world-development-indicators/the-world-by-income-and-region.html

World Bank. (2023a). *Country classification: World bank country and lending groups.* https://datahelpdesk.worldbank.org/knowledgebase/articles/906519-world-bank-country-and-lending-groups

World Bank. (2023b). *Gross national income (GNI) per capita, Atlas method (current US$): World Bank national accounts data, and Organisation for Economic Co-operation and Development (OECD) national accounts data files.* https://data.worldbank.org/indicator/NY.GNP.PCAP.CD

World Health Organization (WHO). (2022, October 1). *Ageing and health: Key facts*https://www.who.int/news-room/fact-sheets/detail/ageing-and-health

World Health Organization (WHO). (n.d.-a) *WHO: Data portal.* https://platform.who.int/data/maternal-newborn-child-adolescent-ageing/indicator-explorer-new/mca/number-of-persons-aged-over-60-years-or-over-(thousands)

World Health Organization (WHO). (n.d.-b). *Ageing-demographics. Data portal: Number of persons aged 60 years or over (thousands).* Retrieved February 22, 2023 from, https://platform.who.int/data/maternal-newborn-child-adolescent-ageing/ageing-data/ageing---demographics

World Health Organization (WHO). (n.d.-c). *Ageing-demographics. Data portal: Percentage of total population aged 60 years or over.* Retrieved February 22, 2023 from, https://platform.who.int/data/maternal-newborn-child-adolescent-ageing/indicator-explorer-new/mca/percentage-of-total-population-aged-60-years-or-over

World Health Organization (WHO). (n.d.-d). *Ageing-demographics. Data portal: Percentage of total population aged 80 years or over.* Retrieved February 22, 2023 from, https://platform.who.int/data/maternal-newborn-child-adolescent-ageing/indicator-explorer-new/mca/percentage-of-total-population-aged-80-years-or-over

World Health Organization (WHO). (n.d.-e). *Ageing-demographics. Data portal: Percentage of total population aged 60 years or over living in rural and urban areas.* Retrieved February 22, 2023 from, https://platform.who.int/data/maternal-newborn-child-adolescent-ageing/

indicator-explorer-new/mca/percentage-of-older-people-aged-60-or-over-living-in-rural-and-urban-areas

World Health Organization (WHO). (n.d.-f). *WHO MNCAH data portal: World bank income group: Global, high income, low income, lower middle income, upper middle income.* https://platform. who.int/data/maternal-newborn-child-adolescent-ageing-data

Zimmer, Z., & Treleaven, E. (2020). The rise and prominence of skip-generation households in lower- and middle-income countries. *Population and Development Review, 46*(4), 709–33.

Selected Bibliography

Battle, S., & Clarke, P. (2022). Inequities in exposure to neighborhood vulnerability over time: Findings from a national sample of U.S. adults. *Race and Social Problems, 14,* 53–68. https://doi. org/10.1007/s12552-021-09343-2

Bigonnesse, C., & Chaudhury, H. (2021). Ageing in place processes in the neighbourhood environment: A proposed conceptual framework from a capability approach. *European Journal of Ageing, 19,* 63–74. https://dol.org/10.1007/s10433-020-00599-y

Fastame, M. D., Ruiu, M., & Mulas, I. (2021). Mental health and religiosity in the Sardinian blue zone: Life satisfaction and optimism for aging well. *Journal of Religion and Health, 60,* 2450–62. https://doi.org/10.1007/s10943-021-01261-2

Hosseinpoor, A. R., Williams, J. A. S., Itani, L., & Chatterji, S. (2012). Socioeconomic inequality in domains of health: Results from the World Health surveys. *BioMed Central, 12.* http://www. biomedcentral.com/1471-2458/12/198

Lopez-Ortiz, S., Lista, S., Penin-Grandes, S., Pinto-Fraga, J., Valenzuela, P. L., Nistico, R., Emanuele, E., Lucia, A., & Santos-Lozano, A. (2022). Defining and assessing intrinsic capacity in older people: A systematic review and a proposed scoring system. *Ageing Research Reviews, 79.* https://doi.org/10.1016/j.arr.2022.101640.

Poulain, M., Herm, A., Errigo, A., Chrysohoou, C., Legrand, R., Passarino, G., Stazi, M. A., Voutekatis, K. G., Gonos, E. S., Francheschi, C., & Pes, G. M. (2021). Specific features of the oldest old from the longevity blue zones in Ikaria and Sardinia. *Mechanisms of Ageing and Development, 198.* https://doi.org/10.1016/j.mad.2021.111543.

Rapp, T., Ronchetti, J., & Sicsic, J. (2022). Where are populations aging better? A global comparison of healthy aging across Organization for Economic Cooperation and Development countries. *Value in Health, 25*(9): 1520–27. http://creativecommons.org/licenses/by/4.0/

Ruiu, M., Carta, V., Deiana, C., & Fastame, M. C. (2022). Is the Sardinian blue zone the new Shangri-la for mental health? Evidence on depressive symptoms and its correlates in late adult life span. *Aging Clinical and Experimental Research, 34,* 1315–22. https://doi.org/10.1007/s40520-021-02068-7

Williams, J. S., Myleus, A., Chatterji, S., & Valentine, N. (2020). Health systems responsiveness among older adults: Findings from the World Health Organization study on global AGEing and adult health. *Global Public Health, 7,* 999–1015. https://doi.org/10.1080/17441692.2020.1742365

Image Credits

THEORIES AND REFLECTIVE PRACTICE

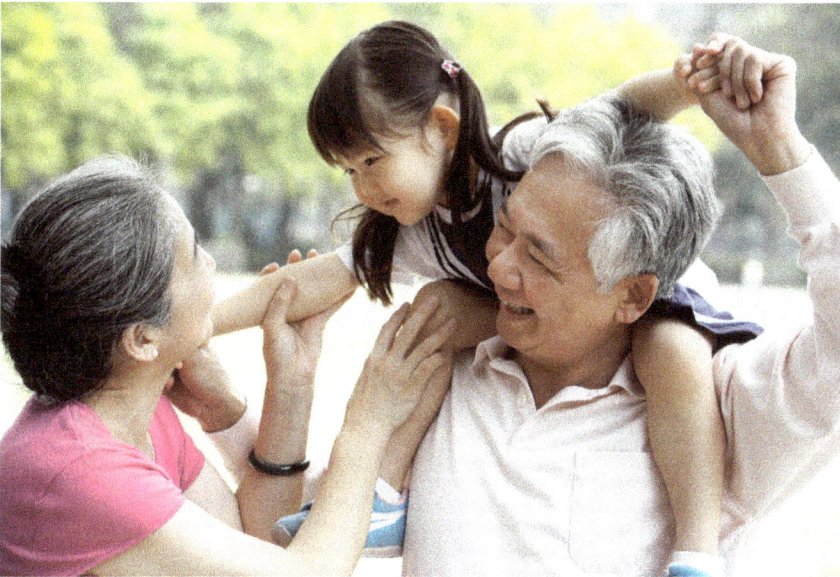

Image 3.1

Overview

This chapter focuses on theories to guide reflective clinical practice and the care of older adults. Theories are organized abstract ideas that explain interrelationships, processes, and end results. Theories derived from these concepts attempt to predict human events. Utilizing, testing, and evaluating theories in health care settings may lead to new insights and modifications or enhancements of the existing ones. It may also lead to discovery of new knowledge, evidence, or information that can be further evaluated for relevance to older adults.

The nursing literature is rich with theories and models, as new knowledge about aging continues to evolve and expand. It is beyond the scope of this chapter to sufficiently address what currently exists in the literature. This presentation is intended to generate ongoing and critical inquiry as the reader encounters additional theories, concepts, and models relevant to the care of older adults. This may enrich understanding and application to practice. Theories inform nursing practice. Furthermore, nursing practice is grounded in evidence. Ultimately, the goal of utilizing theory in practice is to promote effective care and healthy aging.

Outcomes

The learner:

1. Defines the following key terms

    A. Assumption

    B. Concept

    C. Evidence-based practice

    D. Framework

    E. Model

    F. Theory

2. Explains component parts or aspects of a model or theory presented in this chapter

3. Critiques a model or theory as it relates to informing practice and guiding the care of older adults

4. Demonstrates the application of a model or theory in anticipating, guiding, directing, and evaluating care of an older adult

5. Initiates further inquiry into other models and theories and their potential to inform practice and care of aging populations

Introduction

This chapter provides a brief overview of theories and their relevance to the care of aged persons. For some readers this information may be a familiar dialogue, and for other readers this information may be new, or challenging, offering a glimpse into another perspective.

Why Theory?

Theory, for the purposes of this chapter, is derived from a disciplinary philosophy. Nursing is a discipline with its own code of ethics, beliefs and values, standards of practice, unique body of knowledge, and professional governance. Other disciplines (for example, ethics, psychology, anthropology, sociology, biology, physiology) have contributed to nursing philosophy and the development of its theoretical base. A disciplinary philosophy may serve as the basis for development of one's own personal philosophy.

A theory is an abstraction of ideas that attempts to explain realities about the experiences of human beings. Human behavior and actions may be only a surface manifestation of the varied thoughts, feelings, emotions, physicality, and spirituality of the persons health care professionals encounter. Theories help practitioners to understand the world and how humans function within it.

Theories attempt to predict or explain behaviors and relationships and are articulated in coherent, organized, and systematic statements. Symbolically, theories depict realities in relation to observed phenomena. Theories are composed of assumptions and concepts. Assumptions are statements of fact or truth and represent shared beliefs and values. Concepts are terms, classifications, or categorizations describing observed phenomena. Theories are constructed from interrelated assumptions and concepts. As a whole, theories provide insights, guide practice, and inform research. This is important for nurses, caregivers, and health care practitioners, as the intended outcomes of care are to help heal, make whole, and support wellness.

Theory and Research Linkages

Theory is often taught alongside nursing research, as the two are closely intertwined. Nursing research contributes to knowledge and theory development in nursing. The application of a theory in the practice setting affords the opportunity to test the theory and its usefulness with individuals, groups, or populations, also revealing its limitations and opportunities for further research.

Nursing has a rich and well-founded history of theory development, and its contributions to knowledge development continue into the present. Theory has its practical applicability across various roles (leadership and administration, education, clinical practice, and research), health care settings and contexts, and diverse populations.

Nursing scholars, through theory development and understanding of observed phenomena, have integrated beliefs and values about nursing, health, persons (patients/clients/families/groups/populations), and environment. Collectively this is also known as the metaparadigm of the nursing discipline. Theories represent the diverse nature of humankind, the context of the world in which humans live and function, and the philosophical lens of the theorist. Therefore, there is no singular, correct theory. Nonetheless, the reader may find similarities, contrasts, and uniqueness among theories—including grand, mid-range, or micro theories. Early scholars termed their ideas as conceptual frameworks or conceptual models, which may have been a source of confusion among readers. Currently, the works of early scholars such as Neuman (Fawcett & Faust, 2017), Roy (Morrow & Roy, 2022; Roy, 1970, 1980), and followers of Rogers (Wright, 2007; Rogers, 1980) in theory development are referred to as grand theories.

Thinking Conceptually

In one's daily activities, it may be unlikely that thought is devoted to thinking conceptually or theoretically, unless it is intentional or habitual. Nonetheless, the reader is invited to recall a notable situation, experience, or incident related to a health care encounter with an individual or a group. In this exercise:

- Describe the experience or situation.

- Was this an isolated or unique experience? Or a series of experiences and situations?

- What was notable about it?

- Was it an uncomfortable experience? Problematic? Puzzling? Unresolved? In what way?

- Was it a positive or rewarding experience? In what way?

- What did it bring to your awareness? How did it affect you? Were there any insights gained? What were these? Or did you have post-experience insights?

- Were there any identifiable patterns or coincidences?

- How did this encounter affect your perspective or your worldview? Your practice? Subsequent health care encounters with others?

- Describe how this experience generated other related questions or a curiosity to explore further the depth and breadth of such an experience, situation, or observation.

Intentional reflection upon experiences, observations, interactions with others, and surroundings are the seeds of conceptual thinking. Conceptual thinking leads to inductive reasoning from the specific to general, where individual events are observed or experienced and can be combined into a greater whole or a generalized statement. Deductive reasoning moves from a general situation to a specific statement or conclusion. Propositions or hypothesis statements are generated about the relationship between concepts. Concepts or labels given to a phenomena are the basic elements of theory.

Levels of Theoretical Thinking

Higgins and Moore (2000) describe levels of theoretical thinking in nursing. Figure 3.1 illustrates the meta theory or the philosophic inquiry of theory that encompasses the grand, middle-range, and micro-range theories. Exemplars of theories are given at each level, and these are not exhaustive.

Grand theories are highly abstract and describe universal understanding of the discipline of nursing. The language of grand theory may be unfamiliar. Although theories at this level are not highly predictive, there are many examples in the literature in which grand theory has guided research in various areas of practice. Mid-range theories are general, to allow for empirical testing to explain, predict, define, or refine knowledge. Relationships can be measured through quantitative

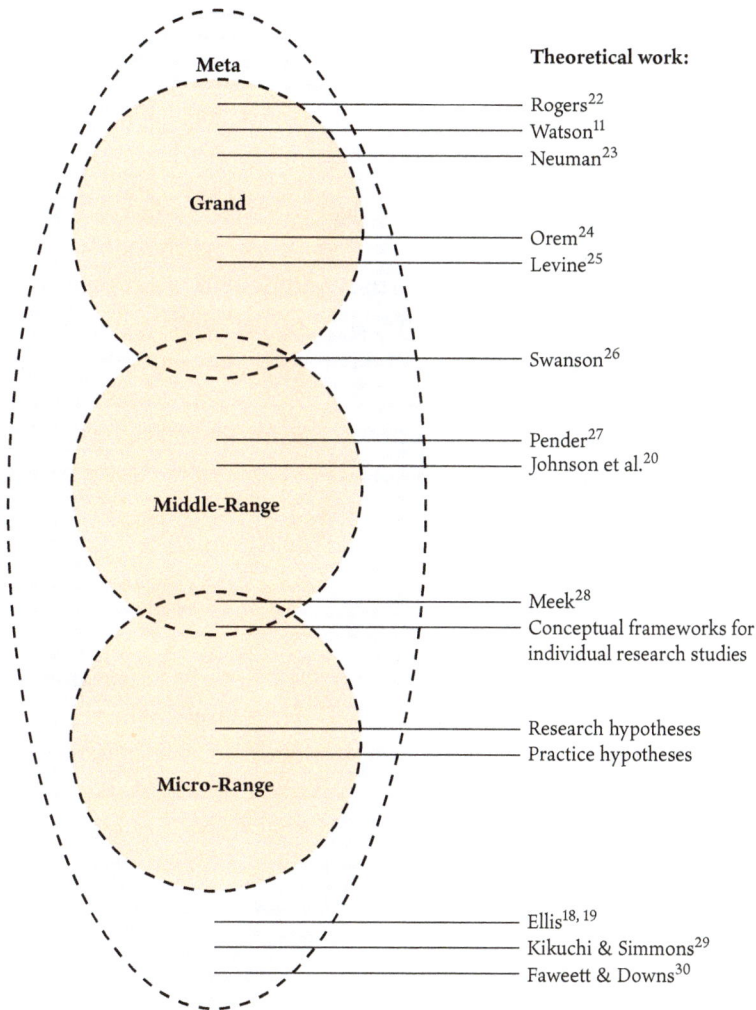

Theoretical work:

Rogers[22]
Watson[11]
Neuman[23]

Orem[24]
Levine[25]

Swanson[26]

Pender[27]
Johnson et al.[20]

Meek[28]
Conceptual frameworks for individual research studies

Research hypotheses
Practice hypotheses

Ellis[18, 19]
Kikuchi & Simmons[29]
Faweett & Downs[30]

Meta

Grand

Middle-Range

Micro-Range

FIGURE 3.1   Levels of Theoretical Thinking

or qualitative research methods. Micro-range theories are highly specific working hypotheses or propositions testing one or two concepts. Applicability of micro-range theories is limited to a single aspect of care.

Evidence-Based Practice (EBP)

Evidence-based practice is a response to the need for continuous knowledge development in nursing and a societal need for care interventions that are effective, feasible, and practical and that result in positive, quality health outcomes.

> Evidence-based practice is a problem solving approach to clinical decision-making within a healthcare organization. EBP integrates the best available scientific evidence with the best available experiential (patient and practitioner) evidence. EBP considers internal and external influences on practice and encourages critical thinking in the judicious application of such evidence in the care of individual patients, a patient population or system. (Dang & Dearholt, 2018, p. 4)

As a problem-solving approach to clinical practice problems, EBP integrates systematic search, critical appraisal, and synthesis of the most relevant and best research, one's own clinical expertise, and patient preferences (Melnyk & Fineout-Overholt, 2011). There are several guidelines and recommendations for the implementation of evidence-based practice in the literature. Practitioners must appraise levels of evidence, or the hierarchy of evidence, for its relevance to patient preferences and values, practitioner experience, health outcomes, and quality of care. Levels of evidence about a study are assigned a value or rating based on established criteria (Burns et al., 2011; Carrington & Love, 2020).

Chapter Summary

This chapter has provided a brief glimpse into theory and its importance to practice and care. Readers have been introduced to basic terms used in theory development. Nursing theory is derived from the philosophy of nursing, values, assumptions, and core beliefs (see Chapter 1). Theory helps to explain situations, relationships, and behaviors. Nurse scholars have developed extensive theories or grand theories, mid-range theories, and micro-theories. Grand theories are highly abstract and all-encompassing of nursing, health, person, and environment concepts and their interrelationships. Mid-range theories are less abstract and lend themselves to testing and measurement with multiple concepts. Micro-range theories are specific, narrow in scope, involve one or two concepts, and may be limited to a specific aspect of care, such as a single treatment or intervention.

Glossary

Assumption: Factual statements or truths representing shared beliefs or values.

Concept: A term (label) that describes a category, classification, or group of phenomena. Concepts are the basic elements of theory. Related concepts form theoretical statements.

Conceptual definition: A comprehensive definition developed by the theorist or researcher that includes associative connotative meanings for research or study purposes. Conceptual definitions provide the basis for operational definitions.

Construct: A construct is similar to a concept except that it is a broader category and includes application of several concepts.

Evidence-based practice: A problem-solving approach to clinical decision-making integrating the best available scientific evidence with the best available experiential (patient and practitioner) evidence, with consideration for internal and external influences, and the judicious application of that evidence.

Framework: A framework is an abstract logical structure of meaning that guides the development of a research study. It is the context in which all variables are considered to bring about desired goals through an action (of the nurse) and received (by a patient). Frameworks are *testable theories* from a conceptual model or from clinical observations (quantitative research) or a worldview consistent with a philosophy (qualitative research; Burns & Grove, 1993; Grove et al., 2015).

Metaparadigm: The philosophy and knowledge of a discipline that includes (a) symbolic generalizations (laws and language of a scientific community), (b) shared commitments to beliefs in models and the methods to create and test such models, (c) shared values that identify what is significant or meaningful to a scientific community, and (d) examples of problems and the methods by which they are solved (Peterson & Bredow, 2004).

Model: A representation of interactions and patterns among concepts. Highly abstract related constructs that explain phenomena of interest, assumptions, and philosophical stance. Another present-day term for highly abstract models is grand nursing theories.

Operational definition: How a specific concept is manipulated through an intervention, or how it is measured.

Research: Systematic inquiry or study undertaken to validate or refine or develop new knowledge within a discipline (Grove et al., 2015).

Qualitative research: A systematic, rigorous approach used to describe experiences and situations from the perspective of the person in the situation. Observed phenomena are the human experiences unique to the individual, time, and context. Qualitative research methods include ethnography, grounded theory, historical, and phenomenological approaches (Grove et al., 2015; Corbin & Strauss, 2015).

Quantitative research: A formal objective, rigorous, systematic process for generating numerical information about the world, it describes new situations, events, or concepts, examines relationships among variables, and determines the effectiveness of treatments or interventions on health outcomes. Quantitative research methods include descriptive, correlational, quasi-experimental, and experimental approaches (Grove et al., 2015).

Theory: An organized, logical set of statements that symbolically communicate reality as a meaningful whole. Theories explain, predict, and describe responses, events, situations, or relationships.

Grand theory: A highly abstract theory revolving around a single phenomenon (examples: adaptation, caring, self-care deficit, systems).

Mid-range theory: A less abstract theory, narrower in scope, with a focus on answering a clinical practice question related to health conditions, family situations, and nursing actions (examples: caregiver stress, pain management, comfort, health promotion).

Micro-theory: A restrictive, particular approach, with respect to time and scope of application; a working proposition to tentatively explain or test health-related interactions or interventions between person and environment.

Variable: This term is more specific than a concept or construct, is narrow in definition, can be measured as a numerical value, and can vary from one instance to another.

References

Burns, N., & Grove, S. K. (1993). *The practice of nursing research: Conduct, critique, & utilization* (2nd ed.). Saunders.

Burns, P. B., Rohrich, R. J., & Chung, K. C. (2011). The levels of evidence and their role in evidence-based medicine. *Plastic Reconstructive Surgery, 128*(1), 305–10. https://doi.10.1097/PRS.0b013e 318219c171

Carrington, J. M., & Love, R. (2020). Development of an innovative tool to appraise big data for best evidence. *Worldviews on Evidence-based Nursing, 17*(4), 269–74.

Corbin, J., & Strauss, A. (2015). *Basics of qualitative research: Techniques and procedures for developing grounded theory* (4th ed.). Sage.

Dang, D., & Dearholt, S. L. (2018). *John Hopkins nursing evidence-based practice: Model and guidelines* (3rd ed.). John Hopkins University School of Nursing.

Fawcett, J., & Foust, J. B. (2017). Optimal aging: A Neuman systems model perspective. *Nursing Science Quarterly, 30*(3), 269–76. https://doi:10.1177/0894318417708413

Higgins, P. A. & Moore, S. M. (2000). Levels of theoretical thinking. *Nursing Outlook, 48,* 179–83. https://doi.10.1067/mno.2000.105248

Grove, S. K., Gray, J. R., & Burns, N. (2015). *Understanding nursing research: Building an evidence-based practice* (6th ed.). Elsevier.

Melnyk, B.M. & Fineout-Overholt, E. (2011). *Evidence-based practice in nursing and health care* (2nd ed.). Wolters Kluwer, Lippincott William & Wilkins

Morrow, M. R., & Roy, C. (2022). A nurse theorist's life of providence: A dialogue with sister Callista Roy. *Nursing Science Quarterly, 35*(3), 311–14. https://doi:10.1177/09843184221092439

Neuman, B., & Fawcett, J. (2012). Thoughts about the Neuman systems model: A dialogue. *Nursing Science Quarterly, 25*(4), 374–76. https://doi.10.1177/0894318412457055

Peterson, S. J., & Bredow, T. S. (2004). *Middle range theories: Application to nursing research.* Lippincott Williams & Wilkins.

Rogers, M. (1980). Nursing: A science of unitary man. In J. P. Riehl & C. Roy (Eds.), *Conceptual models for nursing practice* (2nd ed.; pp. 329–337). Appleton-Century Crofts.

Roy, C. (1970). Adaptation: A conceptual framework for nursing. *Nursing Outlook, 18*(3), 43–45.

Roy, C. (1980). The Roy adaptation model. In J. P. Riehl & C. Roy (Eds.), *Conceptual models for nursing practice* (2nd ed.; pp. 179–188). Appleton-Century Crofts.

Wright, B. W. (2007). Evolution of Rogers science of unitary human beings: 21st century reflections. *Nursing Science Quarterly, 20*(1), 64–67. https://doi:10.1177/0894318406296295

Selected Bibliography

Concept Analysis:

Patrician, P. A., Bakerjian, D., Billings, R., Chenot, T., Hooper, V., Johnson, C. S., & Sables-Baus, S. (2022). Nurse well-being: A concept analysis. *Nursing Outlook, 70*(4), 639–50. https://doi.org/10.1016/j.outlook.2022.03.014

Walker, L., & Avant, K. C. (2011). Concept analysis. In Walker, L., & Avant, K. C. (Eds.), *Strategies for theory construction in nursing* (5th ed; pp. 163–86). Prentice Hall.

Evidence-Based Practice:

Caulfield, E. V., & Valcourt, M. P. (2021). How to critically appraise a research article for evidence-based practice. *International Journal of Safe Patient Handling and Mobility, 11*(2), 100–107.

Gilmartin, M. J. (2023). An evidence-based change management model to guide NICHE implementation efforts. *Geriatric Nursing, 49*, 212–15.

Gorsuch, P. F., Ford, L. G., Thomas, B. K., Melnyk, B. M., & Connor, L. (2020). Impact of a formal educational skill-building program based on the ARCC model to enhance evidence-based practice competency in nurse teams. *Worldviews on Evidence-Based Nursing, 17*(4), 258–68.

Presseau, J., Kasperavicius, D., Rodrigues, I. B., Braimoh, J., Chambers, A., Etherington, C., Giangregorio, L., Gibbs, J. C., Giguere, A., Graham, I. D., Hankivsky, O., Hoens, A. M., Holroyd-Leduc, J., Kelly, C., Moore, J. E., Ponzano, M., Sharma, M., Sibley, K. M., & Straus, S. (2022). Selecting implementation models, theories, and frameworks in which to integrate intersectional approaches. *BioMed Central Medical Research Methodology, 22*, 1–13. https://doi.org/10.1186/s12874-022-01682-x

Speroni, K. G., McLaughlin, M. K., & Friesen, M. A. (2020). Use of evidence-based practice models and research findings in magnet-designated hospitals across the United States: National survey results. *Worldviews on Evidence-Based Nursing, 17*(2), 98–107.

Tucker, S., McNett, M., Melnyk, B. M., Hanrahan, I., Hunter, S. C., Kim, B., Cullen, L., & Kitson, A. (2021). Implementation science: Application of evidence-based practice models to improve healthcare quality. *Worldviews on Evidence-Based Nursing, 18*(2), 76–84.

Mid-Range Theory:

Meleis, A. (1997). *Theoretical nursing: Development and progress* (3rd ed.). Lippincott.

Rosa, W. E., Koithan, M., Kreitzer, M. J., Manjrekar, P., Meleis, A. I., Mukamana, D., Ray, A., & Watson, J. (2020). Nursing theory in the quest for the sustainable development goals. *Nursing Science Quarterly, 33*(2), 178–82. https://doi:org/10.1177/0894318420903495

Nurse Theorists:

LEININGER, MADELEINE

Clarke, P. N., McFarland, M. R., Andrews, M. M., & Leininger, M. (2009). Caring: Some reflections on the impact of the culture care theory by McFarland & Andrews and a conversation with Leininger. *Nursing Science Quarterly, 22*(3), 233–39. https://doi:10.1177/0894318409337020

McFarland, M. R. ,& Wehbe-Alamah, H. B. (2015). *Leininger's culture care diversity and universality: A worldwide nursing theory* (3rd ed.). Jones & Bartlett.

McFarland, M. R. & Wehbe-Alamah, H. B. (2019). Leininger's theory of culture care diversity and universality: An overview with a historical retrospective and a view toward the future. *Journal of Transcultural Nursing, 30*(6), 540–57. https://doi.org10.1177/1043659619867134

Nelson, J. (2006). Madeleine Leininger's culture care theory: The theory of culture care diversity and universality. *International Journal for Human Caring, 10*(4), 50–54.

NEUMAN, BETTY

Angosta, A., Ceria-Ulep, C. D., & Tse, A. M. (2014). Care delivery for Filipino Americans using the Neuman systems model. *Nursing Science Quarterly, 27*(2), 142–48. https://doi:10.1177/0894318 414522605

Basogul, C., & Buldukoglu, K. (2020). Neuman systems model with depressed patients: A randomized controlled trial. *Nursing Science Quarterly, 33*(2), 148–58. https://doi:10,11770894 318419898172

Demir, G. (2018, September–December). The impact of Neuman systems model in reducing care burden on primary caregivers of dementia patients. *International Journal of Caring Sciences, 11*(3). 1849–58.

Eustace, R. W. (2022). A theory of family health: A Neuman's systems perspective. *Nursing Science Quarterly, 35*(1), 101–10. https://doi:10.1177/08943184211051365

McDowell, B. M., Beckman, S., & Fawcett, J. (2023). Created environment: Evolution of a Neuman systems model concept. *Nursing Science Quarterly, 36*(1), 89–91. https://doi:10. 1177/08943184221131975

Vanaki, Z., & Hossein, R. (2020). Application of Betty Neuman system theory in management of pressure injury in patients following stroke. *MedSurg Nursing, 29*(2), 129–33.

NEWMAN, MARGARET

Brown, J. W., Chen, S.-L., Mitchell, C., & Province, A. (2007). Help-seeking by older husbands caring for wives with dementia. *Journal of Advanced Nursing, 59*(4), 352–60. https://doi.10.1111/ j.13652648.2007.04290.x

Endo, E. (2016). Margaret Newman's theory of health as expanding consciousness and a nursing intervention from a unitary perspective. *Asia Pacific Journal of Oncology Nursing, 4*(1), 50–52.

Imaizumi, S., Honda, A., Fujiwara, Y., Iio, Y. (2021). Caring partnership within Newman's theory of health as expanding consciousness: Aiming for patients to find meaning in their treatment experiences. *Asia Pacific Journal of Oncology Nursing, 8*(6), 725–31.

Smith, M. C. (2011). Integrative review of research related to Margaret Newman's theory of health as expanding consciousness. *Nursing Science Quarterly, 24*(3), 256–72. https://doi:10.1177/08943 18411409421

Yang, A., Xiong, D., Vang, E., & Pharris, M. D. (2009). Hmong American women living with diabetes. *Journal of Nursing Scholarship, 41*(2), 139–48. https://doi.10.1111/j1547-5069, 2009.01265.x

OREM, DOROTHEA

Gumbs, J. (2020). Orem's select basic conditioning factors and health promoting self-care behaviors among African American women with type 2 diabetes. *Journal of Cultural Diversity, 27*(2), 47–52.

Hartweg, D. L. (1991). *Dorothea Orem Self-care deficit theory: Notes of nursing theories.* Sage.

Hartweg, D. L., & Metcalfe, S. A. (2022). Orem's self-care deficit nursing theory: Relevance and need for refinement. *Nursing Science Quarterly, 35*(1), 70–76. https://doi:10.1177/08943184211 051369

Hartweg, D. L., & Pickens, J. (2016). A concept analysis of normalcy within Orem's self-care deficit nursing theory. *Self-Care, Dependent-Care & Nursing, 22*(1), 4–13.

Reiszadeh, I., Abolhassani, S., Masoudi, R., & Kheiri, S. (2022). The effect of self-care program based on the Orem self-care model on fatigue and quality of life in patients with COPD. *Journal of Nursing and Midwifery Sciences, 9*(4), 241–48.

Tanaka, M. (2022). Orem's nursing self-care deficit theory: A theoretical analysis focusing on its philosophical and sociological foundation. *Nursing Forum, 57,* 480–85. https://doi:10.1111/nuf.12696

PURNELL, LARRY

Purnell, L. (2000). A description of the Purnell model for cultural competence. *Journal of Transcultural Nursing, 11*(1), 40–46.

Purnell, L. (2002). The Purnell model for cultural competence. *Journal of Transcultural Nursing, 13*(3), 193–96.

Purnell, L. (2013). *Transcultural health care: A culturally competent approach* (4th ed.). F.A. Davis.

WATSON, JEAN

Costello, M., & Barron, A. M. (2017). Teaching compassion: Incorporating Jean Watson's caritas processes into a care at the end of life course for senior nursing students. *International Journal of Caring Sciences, 10*(3), 1113–17.

Goldberg, L., Rosenburg, N., & Watson, J. (2018). Rendering LGBTQ+ visible in nursing. *Journal of Holistic Nursing, 36*(1), 262–71. https://doi.org/10.1177/0898010117715141

Gunawan, J., Aungsuroch, Y., Watson, J., & Marzilli, C. (2022). Nursing administration: Watson's theory of human caring. *Nursing Science Quarterly, 35*(2), 235–43. https://doi.org/10.1177/089431

Hills, M., Watson, J., & Cara, C. (2021). *Creating a caring science curriculum: A relational emancipatory pedagogy for nursing* (2nd ed.). Springer.

Morrow, M. R., & Watson, J. (2022). Nursing is the light in institutional darkness: A dialogue with Dr. Jean Watson. *Nursing Science Quarterly, 35*(1), 35–40. https://doi:10.1177/0894318 4211051349

Revels, A., Goldberg, L., & Watson, J. (2016). Caring science: A theoretical framework for palliative care in the emergency department. *International Journal for Human Caring, 20*(4), 206–11.

Rossillo, K., Norman, V., Wickman, J., & Winokur, M. (2020). Caritas education: Theory to practice. *International Journal for Human Caring, 24*(2), 106–20.

Watson, J. (2022). Watson's view of *Nursing Science Quarterly*'s 35th anniversary. *Nursing Science Quarterly, 35*(1), 67–69. https://doi:10.1177/08943184211051366

Watson, J., Porter-O'Grady, T., Horton-Deutsch, S., & Malloch, K. (2018). Quantum caring leadership: Integrating quantum leadership with caring science. *Nursing Science Quarterly, 31*(3), 253–58. https://doi:10.1177/0894318418774893

Websites

Betty Neuman Systems Theory. (n.d.). *Core concepts of the Betty Neuman's the systems model.* https://nurseslabs.com/betty-neuman-systems-model-nursing-theory/

Center for Evidence-Based Practice. (n.d.). *Evidence-based practice model & tools.* https://www.hopkinsmedicine.org/evidence-based-practice/model-tools.html

University of San Diego (USD) Hahn School of Nursing and Health Science. (n.d.). *Nursing theory and research: A collection of nursing theory from around the world.* https://www.sandiego.edu/nursing/research/nursing-theory-research.php

Watson Caring Science Institute. (n.d.). *Watson's caring science & human caring theory.* https://www.watsoncaringscience.org/jean-bio/caring-science-theory/

Videos

Engel, M. (2021, September 21). *Conversations in healthcare. Dr. Jean Watson: Nursing, humanity, and the circle of life-compassion and courage-episode 3*[Video]. YouTube. https://www.youtube.com/watch?v=5GZO2kU3EtY

Home Care of Rochester. (2008). *Dr. Madeleine Leininger interview, part 1*[Video]. YouTube. https://www.youtube.com/watch?v=a4GTo_uthZQ

Home Care of Rochester. (2008). *Dr. Madeleine Leininger interview, part 2*[Video]. YouTube. https://www.youtube.com/watch?v=6xchWCgeMM4

Watson, J. (2018). *10 Caritas processes*[Video]. Vimeo. https://vimeo.com/239311060

Watson, J. (2020). *Caring science and integrative nursing*[Video]. Vimeo. https://vimeo.com/405053163

Watson, J. (2020). *Clinical practice of human caring (with Spanish subtitles)*[Video]. Vimeo. https://vimeo.com/370531025

Image Credits

CULTURE AND AGING

Overview

Culture is defined as those shared beliefs, values, and boundaries in which persons operate to feel a sense of belonging to a group based on values shared by the group. In opposition to ethnocentrism, understanding the culture of another fosters empathy, suspends judgment, and broadens one's worldview. Many communities with aging populations are increasingly diverse. Therefore, nurses must possess knowledge, skills, and abilities to provide interculturally sensitive, safe, and competent care from a perspective of cultural humility. Furthermore, the ANA Code of Ethics, as discussed in Chapter 1, gives the following injunction: "The nurse in all professional relationships, practices with compassion and respect for the inherent dignity, worth, and uniqueness of every individual, unrestricted by considerations of social or economic status, personal attributes, or the nature of health problems."

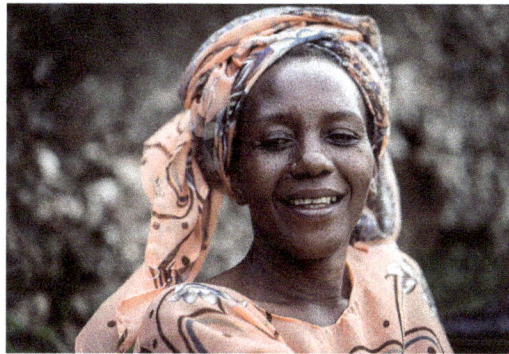

Outcomes

The learner:

1. Defines the following terms

   A. Ethnocentrism

   B. Stereotyping

   C. Bias

   D. Intersectionality

   E. Culture

      a. Cultural sensitivity

      b. Cultural humility

      c. Cultural competence

   F. Worldview

      a. Etic

      b. Emic

   G. Diversity

   H. Transcultural nursing

2. Seeks and negotiates shared understanding through communication (verbal and nonverbal) in the context of cultural differences

3. Develops meaningful interactions with culturally diverse older adults by suspending judgment and valuing interactions with different others

Introduction

Culture is the shared and learned values and beliefs of a group. Cultural beliefs and values are expressed in behaviors, emotions, language, and communication. Broad definitions of culture extend to organizations or institutions that ascribe to a set of shared attitudes, values, goals, and practices. It is also a pattern of human knowledge, belief, and behavior that depends on the capacity for learning and transmitting knowledge to succeeding generations.

Dimensions of culture are multifaceted, complex, and diverse. With relevance to healthy aging, the reader is gently pushed toward exploration and discovery as new knowledge in human science emerges. Lifelong learning and a willingness to engage in dialogue and relationships with diverse older adults can lead to an enriched cultural understanding of others.

Beyond Outward Characteristics

Beyond outward characteristics of ethnicity, dress, and food, culture shapes one's worldview about wellness, illness, health beliefs, and health decision-making. World-view is the lens through which one perceives and understands the world. It extends to orientation toward time and orientation toward self, family, gender roles, and communication. Communication may be nuanced and indirect or explicit and direct. Decisions may be individual or collective. Another way in which culture is reflected is the extent to which there is greater or lesser reliance on social environmental cues—context dependent or context independent, respectively.

Tertiary, secondary, and *primary* are terms used to describe levels of culture. At the tertiary level, culture is publicly manifested to outsiders through manner of dress, cuisine, and special events or festivals. At the secondary level, members of a group have and know underlying rules and assumptions that are not often communicated or shared with outsiders. The primary levels of culture are the implicit rules known and followed by a group and are the deepest level of culture and rarely shared with outsiders.

Cultural Competence, Humility, and Sensitivity

Cultural competence comprises knowing and action, or actionable knowledge. Competence is acquired through learning. It is the ability to act with awareness and understanding of the patient's situation in the context of their beliefs, values, and customs, along with their social and political worldview.

The term "cultural competence" has been criticized as it implies a reduction to technical skills and because of its association within the stereotypical limits of ethnicity, nationality, and language of patients (Kleinman & Benson, 2006). Hence, health care institutions and health care providers may unknowingly be perpetrators of stigma, bias, and health care disparities through the medicalization of problems when patients seek care. Kleinman & Benson (2006) offer an explanatory model approach to understanding the patient's perceptions (see Table 4.1). Berlin and Fowkes (1983) have been early proponents of a cross-cultural communication process. Foremost in these guidelines is that of listening (see Table 4.2), as effective planning cannot occur without this.

TABLE 4.1 The Explanatory Models Approach

- What do you call this problem?

- What do you believe is the cause of the problem?

- What course do you expect it to take? How serious is it?

- What do you think this problem does inside your body?

- How does it affect your body and your mind?

- What do you fear most about this condition?

- What do you fear most about the treatment?

Source: Anthropology in the clinic: The problem with cultural competency and how to fix it (Kleinman & Benson, 2006).

TABLE 4.2 Guidelines for Health Practitioners: LEARN

L *Listen* with sympathy and understanding to the patient's perception of the problem.

- What do you feel may be causing your problem?

- How do you feel the illness is affecting you?

- What do you feel might be of benefit?

E *Explain*

- Explain or communicate the diagnosis from a "Western medicine" or biomedical perspective.

- Have a strategy and convey the strategy to the patient.

A *Acknowledge*

- Acknowledge and integrate the patient's and the provider's explanatory models.

- Understand and resolve areas of agreement and conflict. Understanding involves bridging the conceptual gap between different belief systems.

R *Recommend*

- Develop a treatment plan using the patient's and provider's explanatory model.

- Include appropriate culturally relevant approaches. Patient involvement is crucial.

N *Negotiate*

- It is important to understand the patient's perspective and communicate the provider's perspective.

- Utilize options from several disciplines in creating a patient-provider partnership in decision-making.

Modified from source: A teaching framework for cross-cultural health care: Application in family practice (Berlin & Fowkes, 1983).

Cultures are diverse and multifaceted. One realizes there are limitations in possessing comprehensive knowledge of all cultures and that *multiple realities exist*. Openness to continuous learning and understanding of another's context and situation fosters competence. For example, persons who ascribe to a particular faith may have dietary restrictions or are steadfast in their beliefs about not accepting certain medical treatment and interventions. The nurse, having cultural knowledge and awareness of the patient's faith or practices, strives to learn more by asking and accommodating to ensure culturally congruent care. The nurse may ask, "Which spiritual practices do you honor throughout the day?" rather than "What is your religion?" "Are there beliefs or customs that influence your food choices?" rather than "Are there foods you do not eat?" Another solicitation may be "Tell me more about faith beliefs that may influence your decision to consent or not consent to medications, treatments, or procedures." Actionable knowledge of another's culture allows for openness and accommodation of patient preferences. Just as nursing knowledge and science continue to grow and evolve, so does the continuous development of cultural competence in one's practice. As culture is dynamic, so is the lifelong professional development toward cultural competence.

Often in nursing practice, little is taken into account of the culture and worldview of the health care provider and those systems and infrastructures of care the patient encounters. Furthermore, health care provider assumptions or stereotypes about the patient can result in undesirable negative outcomes.

It is often thought that routine care and treatment interventions will be fully accepted, only to be met with resistance, refusal, or non-consent. This situation occurs because the patient has not been consulted or given knowledge needed to make an informed decision. From a Western standpoint, health assessments may be conducted in a manner that is clipped, brisk, and impersonal. Acquisition of information in this manner may seem beneficial to the nurse or health care provider, but it is impractical and of very little use if it ignores the patient's situation, context, and worldview. The purpose of an initial patient assessment is to acquire information to individualize care, not merely to meet institutional policy requirements for timely documentation. Using assessment information effectively to accommodate person-centered and culturally congruent care is cultural competence.

The concept of cultural humility allows for infinite opportunities for growth and understanding. Cultural humility is the stance or attitude in health care interactions whereby the nurse or health care provider recognizes and acknowledges that the individual patient is the expert of their own life, cultural background, and experience. Cultural humility also requires internal examination of one's own biases. This stance of cultural humility is one of respect, which in turn facilitates cultural sensitivity. Cultural sensitivity tailors communication, care, and interventions to the individual person seeking care. At the same time, the nurse or health care provider focuses attention on the patient's narrative and sets aside personal biases and assumptions held about another (see Table 4.1).

Cultural humility and sensitivity invite the exploration of another's worldview on health and well-being, illness causation, Indigenous or traditional practices across the life course, and end of life experience. Culturally congruent care, then, is care based on knowledge, actions, and decisions used in sensitive, appropriate, and meaningful ways befitting cultural values and beliefs for health, illness prevention, disability, and end of life care (see Figure 4.1).

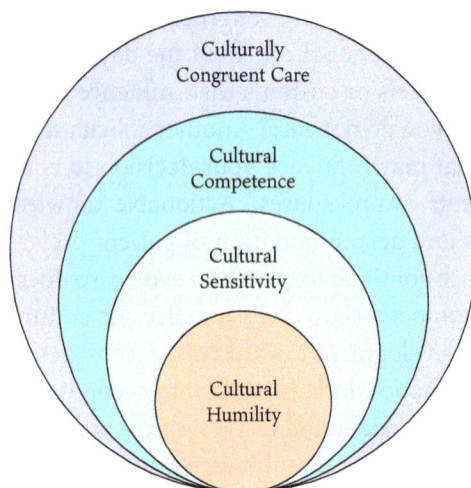

FIGURE 4.1   Cultural humility is the core of every health care encounter—individual patient, family, group, or community. Cultural humility brings about awareness and sensitivity to other worldviews. With cultural humility and sensitivity as the basis for understanding, the nurse seeks further knowledge through learning or education and experiences. Humility, sensitivity, and competence foster culturally congruent care.

Transcultural Nursing

Cultural competence, humility, and sensitivity facilitate culturally congruent care. These are essential to transcultural nursing practice. Transcultural nursing is the ability to provide compassionate, wholistic, relevant, effective care within dynamic cultural contexts to diverse persons, groups, and communities, inclusive of their environmental, economic, geographic, and sociopolitical situations, and beliefs and values (Douglas & Pacquiao, 2010).

Leininger's Theory of Culture Care Diversity and Universality (Leininger, 2006) is widely recognized as the theoretical basis for transcultural nursing practice. Major assumptions underlying the theory are as follows:

1. Care is the central unifying focus of nursing.

2. Humanistic and scientific care is essential to growth and well-being.

3. Caring is essential to curing, and both are necessary and relevant.

4. Culture care guides the researcher in discovering and explaining health and wellbeing.

5. Culture care expressions, meanings, and patterns are diverse and universal among cultures.

6. Culture care is influenced by and embedded in worldview and socio-structural, historical, and environmental contexts.

7. Cultures have both generic (emic) and professional (etic) care for culturally congruent practices.

8. Culturally congruent and therapeutic care is that which occurs when values, beliefs, care expressions, and care patterns are known and used in an appropriate, sensitive, and meaningful manner with persons of diverse or similar cultures.

9. Modes of care (decisions and actions) provide therapeutic ways to help diverse cultures.

10. Qualitative research paradigms are important in the discovery of culture care knowledge and practices. Specifically, ethnonursing methodology facilitates discovery utilizing qualitative evaluative criteria (credibility, confirmability, meaning-in-context, recurrent patterning, saturation, and transferability).

11. Transcultural nursing seeks to attain and maintain culturally congruent care.

Major concepts embedded within Leininger's theory are further defined as follows:

1. Care and caring are those actions, attitudes, and practices to help with healing and well-being; care acknowledges and incorporates cultural and symbolic meanings (protection, respect, presence).

2. Culture guides decisions and actions in patterned ways, intergenerationally, over time, and in different locations.

3. Social structure factors directly or indirectly influence health and well-being.

4. Modes of care are decisions and actions (preservation-maintenance, accommodation-negotiation, repatterning-restructuring) that promote culturally congruent care for health, well-being, and end of life care.

Leininger's Sunrise Enabler to Discover Culture Care

The Sunrise Enabler to Discover Culture Care (Leininger, 2006) is a visual model depicting how the Theory of Culture Care Diversity and Universality may be utilized across diverse cultures and contexts (see Figure 4.2). The Sunrise Enabler embraces holism, multiple factors that constitute environmental context, language and ethnohistory, and cultural and socio-structural dimensions. In totality, these form a worldview.

At the very core of the Enabler are care expressions, patterns, and practices of health, illness, and death. Arising above this core are context, language, and ethnohistory. These are multiple factors that influence the core care expressions, patterns, and practices. The double-headed arrows throughout the model represent interactivity and the dynamic nature of the model. The three interlinking circles acknowledge care practices both emic (generic, folk care), and etic (nursing care and cure) practices.

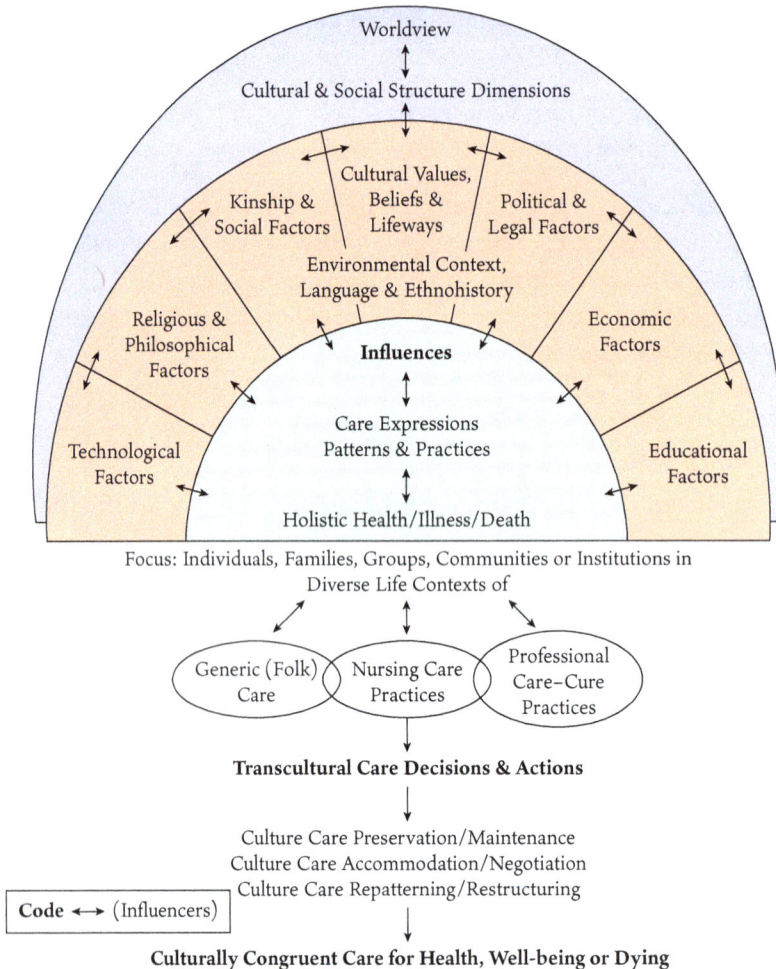

FIGURE 4.2   Leininger's Sunrise Enabler to Discover Culture Care

Unique to the Enabler are the three action-decision care modes of culture care (Leininger & McFarland, 2006):

- Preservation-maintenance: assistive, supportive, facilitative acts that preserve or maintain care beliefs and values;

- Accommodation-negotiation: care actions or decisions that help adapt or negotiate for congruent, safe, effective care;

- Repatterning-restructuring: professional actions and mutual decisions to help reorder, change, modify, or restructure lifeways and institutions for better patterns, practices, or outcomes.

The nurse has a key role in each of the action-decision care modes. Observation, participation, reflection, and confirmation are necessary in culture care, as it also is in the conduct of qualitative nursing research. The Sunrise Enabler integrates the ideas introduced by previously mentioned authors and their work. It is useful across diverse cultures, contexts, settings, time, and life cycles.

Culture Care and Older Adults

Older adults have a lifetime of lived experiences and multifaceted expressions, patterns, and practices of care. They have a unique ethnohistory influenced by many sociocultural factors that informs their worldview. Aging may be viewed differently within various cultures. Family position, social support, independence, self-sufficiency, work, and gender roles have their own meaning and significance as people age. Therefore, cultural knowledge, sensitivity, and congruent care are paramount in working with and caring for older adults.

As previously discussed, Leininger's Sunrise Enabler readily facilitates a culture care assessment in many dimensions. Essential precursors to a culture care assessment are mutual trust and respect. The presence of mutual trust and respect may occur within the brief span of the health care provider-patient encounter or interaction, or over a lengthier period of time. Without trust or respect, further culture care discovery, care decisions and actions, and particularly negotiation or restructuring will be ineffective at best. The nurse or health care provider must be sensitive to the use of forms of address when communicating with patients, as well as their use of gestures and language, including medical jargon or slang, which may be misunderstood. The manner or tone in which the nurse or health care provider elicits information may influence the outcome of the interaction. How one is positioned relative to the patient warrants consideration. Being at eye level with the patient, rather than towering over the patient, may seem less authoritative or threatening. Having knowledge of cultural customs or traditions demonstrates appreciation and respect of the other. For example, in Cambodian culture, it is disrespectful to point the soles of one's feet toward another while seated on the floor during temple ceremonies or prayers.

In addition to the frameworks proposed by Kleinman (2006) and Berlin and Fowkes (1983), the nurse can utilize culture care assessment as a dialogue of discovery. Open-ended questions lend themselves to this, notwithstanding any life-threatening emergencies or urgencies of the patient's situation (see Table 4.3; Exemplar 1).

TABLE 4.3 Supplementary Guidelines and Question Examples: The Nurse-Patient Encounter

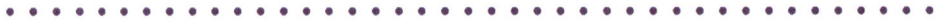

• •

Introduce yourself

- Ask the patient how they would like to be addressed, including preferred pronouns or titles.
- Note that the gender of the nurse or health care provider may matter to the patient; if this is a concern, seek out another health care provider of the patient's preferred gender, make introductions, and provide a thorough report to also include the patient's perspective on care and treatment.
- Position yourself at eye level with the patient, as equals.

Elicit the patient's health care concerns or their story about how they came to seek care:

- "How may I help?"
- "What concerns you the most at this time?"
- "Please tell me more about … "
- "How often does this happen?"
- "Can you please describe further … ?"
- "Please give me an example …"
- "Tell me what you are doing when this happens."
- "What do you do to stay well?"
- "What do you do when you are ill?"
- "Who decides the care and treatment you should receive?"
- "Are there others who help you in making a decision about the care and treatment you should receive?"
- "How does your current condition or situation affect you?"
- "How does your current circumstance affect your daily life?"
- "How are others affected by your current situation?"

Accurately restate the patient's account from their perspective; validate and confirm their perceptions.

- "As I understand … "
- "This is what you have told me …"
- "Is this correct … ?"
- "If I misunderstood, please correct me …"

During the physical assessment, ask permission first and maintain dignity by draping, thereby exposing only the area that is being assessed. Explain why the assessment is important. Explain noninvasive equipment that may be used and what it will do.

Ask permission to remove accessory items that are worn if these interfere with the physical assessments. These items may have spiritual or religious significance to the individual wearing them.

- "May I listen to your breathing?"
- "I am going to place this instrument (stethoscope) on different parts of your chest to listen to your breathing."
- "I will place this device on your fingertip, which will tell me about your pulse (or how fast your heart is beating) and your temperature."

Offer an explanation (diagnosis, hypothesis) of what you think is occurring. Be cognizant that Western biomedical concepts or diseases and terms used to describe such may be unfamiliar, or there may be no terms or language to describe such in the patient's culture. Convey your concerns and a plan. Elicit the patient's concerns about the plan. Integrate the patient's approaches in the plan.

Provide simple explanations, using modes of communication meaningful to the patient—drawings, animations, models, medical interpreters.

- "This is what I think is happening ..."
- "What do you think is happening?"
- "What do you think should be done?"
- "What worries you about ... ?"
- "This is what I have found ... and it means that ..."

Provide thorough and accurate information, with explanation in a manner the patient comprehends. The patient makes an *informed decision*, including the right to *refuse* or *change* their course of action.

- "How can we work together to bring you back to wellness or health?"
- "What do you fear about the care or treatment?"
- "What do you want done, or not done?"
- "What would prevent you from participating in the care or treatment?"
- "What would you like to see happen?"
- "What are the most important results that should happen from the care or treatment?"
- "Who else should help?"

Follow-through, reliability, and ongoing communication throughout the nurse-patient encounter, whether brief or over time, is paramount to sustaining mutual trust and respect. This is a professional expectation.

- Keep your word, no matter how trivial or major the action.
- Truthfully explain an untoward or unexpected course of events.
- Use sensitivity in communicating adverse news; assistance may be needed from a family member or the family spokesperson.
- Seek realistic, feasible, and appropriate care and treatment alternatives that cause no undue harm or suffering; these may be Western/biomedical, Indigenous care or treatments, or both.

Language, the vehicle of communication, understanding, and shared meaning are central to the transmission of values, human interactions, and experiences. It is through language (verbal and nonverbal) within the health care encounter that nurse and patient, or caregiver and care recipient, engage in exchange of information and a process of gathering evidence to arrive at a culturally congruent plan of care and therapeutic outcomes. It is the right of patients to have culturally and linguistically appropriate services.

National Culturally and Linguistically Appropriate Standards (CLAS)

The United States Department of Health and Human Services (USDHHS) established national Culturally and Linguistically Appropriate Standards (CLAS) for communication and language assistance. Given the language diversity and demographic shifts in many communities, the CLAS "provide effective, equitable, understandable, and respectful quality care and services that are responsive to diverse cultural health beliefs and practices, preferred languages, health literacy, and other communication needs" (USDHHS, n.d.).

The CLAS ensure, regardless of age, background, status, race, or beliefs, a right to equitable care and that language is no communication barrier. Nonetheless, bias, discrimination, ageism, and stereotyping remain pervasive in society. The emphasis on differences may serve to oppress groups or hinder care. The interaction of multiple forms of discrimination imposed by power, social structures, and inequality, experienced over time, leads to increasing health care disparities and further marginalization of older adults. Crenshaw describes this as intersectionality (NAIS, 2018).

Certified medical interpreters can effectively bridge cross-cultural communication gaps, thereby alleviating problematic health care encounters. Family, relatives, and children, who are often used as interpreters, may have insufficient medical knowledge to accurately interpret the patient's health care issues or their meaning. There may also be sensitive issues that an older adult cannot communicate, or may not wish to communicate, to a health care provider through their children, a well-intended friend, or a relative.

It is important to uphold the requests of the patient for a medical interpreter with respect to gender and spoken language. It may be inappropriate for a female patient to communicate her concerns through a male interpreter, and the same holds true for male patients. Interpreter preferences of non-binary and LGBTQ+ older adults must also be accommodated. Spoken languages may have more than one dialect, and such preferences should also be explored with the patient.

The dynamic of triadic communication between health care provider, patient, and medical interpreter is an extremely important one. The focus of communication is between the nurse or health care provider and the patient. The nurse addresses the patient. The interpreter is the medium through which communication occurs. Ask simple questions, or one question at a time, instead of compound questions. Allow time for the interpreter to ask the question and for the patient to respond. Likewise, the interpreter also needs time to thoughtfully and accurately represent the patient's statements. It is essential that the nurse or other healthcare provider establish and maintain therapeutic communication and rapport with both the patient and the medical interpreter. This fosters trust in the process and the exchange of relevant meaningful information and evidence for quality patient outcomes.

Issues may arise when there is a lengthy exchange between the interpreter and the patient with only a terse reply to the nurse or health care provider about what actually transpired in the communication. It is helpful to confer with the interpreter prior to the patient health care encounter (see Exemplar 2).

Medical interpreters are held to the same ethical standards and legislative mandates of maintaining confidentiality and privacy of patient information as are all direct care providers. The Health Insurance Portability and Accountability Act of 1996 (HIPAA; USDHHS, 2021) established national standards to safeguard patient information. Sensitive and personal information is shared back and forth between the patient and the health care provider through the interpreter. Confidentiality and privacy of patient information is not limited to the verbal encounter during an interaction but also to forms that require the patient's written consent.

The concept of informed consent must be explained clearly in a manner that the patient comprehends and understands to make decisions and take informed action. In addition to the services of an interpreter, a variety of modalities using the patient's language are helpful—infographics, videos, literature, or peer counselors or advocates. Consent forms often use medical and legal terms and complex sentences that may not be easily understood, especially by persons who are English language learners, or who speak English as a second language.

Conceptual equivalence and semantic meaning are vital in the translation of materials for patient use. Back translation is an iterative process that helps ensure conceptual equivalence and semantic meaning. Materials are translated from the host language to the target language, and the same materials are translated back from the target language to the host language. Independent expert interpreters are used in this process (Brislin, 1970).

Health Literacy

Nurses have a professional and ethical responsibility, substantiated in the ANA Code of Ethics, to promote health literacy. The Centers for Disease Control and Prevention (CDC) define personal and organizational health literacy as follows:

- Personal health literacy is the degree to which individuals have the ability to find, understand, and use information and services to inform health-related decisions and actions for themselves and others.

- Organizational health literacy is the degree to which organizations equitably enable individuals to find, understand, and use information and services to inform health-related decisions and actions for themselves and others. (CDC, n.d.)

A professional responsibility in promoting health literacy includes providing guidance and direction in seeking and using valid, reliable evidence and information sources widely available online.

Health literacy allows for effective self-care management. Older adults have the ability and capacity for new learning and adaptation. Many websites include information and health education materials in other languages and in multiple formats to appeal to various learning styles. The use of color, larger font, closed-caption, and written transcripts allows the older adult patient to choose a suitable modality. Health care institutions employ, in addition to interpreters, multilingual health care professionals or cultural health liaisons, who are representative of the ethnic populations in their respective communities.

Chapter Summary

This chapter familiarizes the learner with definitions related to culture and culture care considerations in working with the older adult. Leininger's Sunrise Enabler is an appropriate vehicle for discovering cultural lifeways, patterns, and practices of the older adult. It is universal, as it may be used across cultures, contexts, and situations. Other key factors central to culture and older adults are those of working effectively with medical interpreters and the promotion of health literacy.

Glossary

Bias: A personal inclination or unreasoned judgment toward another.

Culture: Shared and learned values, beliefs of a group; a way of life shared by people in a place or time; knowledge, beliefs, morals, laws, customs; system of shared ideas, concepts, rules, and meanings that underlie a way of life; explicit and implicit guidelines of members of society that guide views, experiences of the world, and behaviors; cultures are complex wholes and never homogeneous.

Cultural competence: "A complex know-act grounded in critical reflection and action, which the health care professional draws upon to provide culturally safe, congruent, and effective care in partnership with individuals, families, and communities living health experiences, and which takes into account the social and political dimensions of care" (Garneau & Pepin, 2015).

Cultural humility: An approach to interpersonal interactions that focuses on respect and lack of superiority toward another individual's cultural background and experience; a committed practice of self-reflection upon one's own implicit biases and assumptions, lifelong learning from patients who are expert in their own lives, recognizing and mitigating power imbalances, and being accountable in serving diverse persons by providing resources, support, infrastructure, and skilled health care providers.

Cultural sensitivity: "Cultural sensitivity is employing one's knowledge, consideration, understanding, respect, and tailoring after realizing awareness of self and others and encountering a diverse group or individual. Cultural sensitivity results in effective communications, effective interventions, and satisfaction" (Foronda, 2008).

Diversity inclusion: Recognizing and valuing all the different characteristics that make one individual or group different from another, including not only race, ethnicity, and gender—the groups that most often come to mind when this term is used—but also age, national origin, religion, disability status, gender identity, sexual orientation, socioeconomic status, education, marital status, language, and physical appearance, as well as different ideas, perspectives, and values.

Ethnocentrism: The belief or attitude that one's own group (ethnicity, nationality) is superior to others; the tendency to comprehend and judge the world from the perspective of one's culture, evaluate other cultures by the standards and practices of one's own cultural group, or view one's own way of life as the only proper or moral way.

Etic: Extrinsic perspective of the cultural outsider, such as health care professionals and researchers and observers.

Emic: Perspective of a cultural insider; lay folks' or Indigenous perspectives on matters such as health and illness, intrinsic and shared cultural distinctions, cultural insider.

Implicit bias: The attitudes or stereotypes that affect a person's understanding, actions, and decisions in an unconscious manner; biases, both favorable and unfavorable, are activated involuntarily and without the person's awareness.

Intersectionality: The complex, cumulative way in which the effects of multiple forms of discrimination (such as racism, sexism, and classism) combine, overlap, or intersect, especially in the experiences of marginalized individuals or groups.

Stereotyping: An oversimplified opinion, prejudiced attitude, or judgment held in common by members of a group toward others; the supposition that all people in a group are alike and share the same values and beliefs; a general and naïve impression of a group based on physical appearance, history, characteristics, or unique aspects of a group.

Transcultural nursing care: The ability to transform care in a manner that is culture-specific and congruent, safe, and beneficial for health, well-being, and healing. Transcultural nursing care also helps diverse people face disabilities and end of life that is assistive, supportive, therapeutic, and culturally sensitive.

Worldview: A conception of the world from one's specific standpoint.

Exemplar 1: Gaining Entre

An exemplar is an actual experience, lived, witnessed, or observed, used to illustrate or model those ideas, actions, or concepts expressed in the chapter.

A mentor had advised me that there was "much work" yet to be done with a refugee community. As a graduate student at the time, I was eager to embark on an area of study that has long held my interests. These interests were influenced by my own cultural experiences, my upbringing, and the community and environment in which I was raised. My immediate focus was obtaining interviewees for a qualitative study.

The community of interest to me was located in Southern California, 45 miles from where I lived at the time. Through my mentor, I was introduced to the director of a nearby social services agency, who with her staff of social workers, translators, administrative personnel, and health care providers, worked closely with a Cambodian community. This tightly knit community consisted of recently resettled individuals, groups, and families. The social services agency provided a vast array of comprehensive services that touched every aspect of daily living in an environment where language, customs, and way of life were foreign to the newly arrived.

"Volunteer," my mentor advised, as a way of getting to know the community. She also referred me to a community liaison whom the community looked up to for referrals, communication, and advice. I did volunteer, met with the director, and expressed my main intent for being there. The director asked me what I was willing to do to help the community. Essentially, I did whatever was asked and whatever was needed—participated in health fairs, taught a weekly life skills course to the staff who worked closely with the community, tutored English, helped supervise young children in after-school programs while their parents worked, drove children to outings to the beach, played jump rope and basketball, helped with fundraising, and attended cultural celebrations (American and Cambodian), weekly temple, and funerals.

During this period, I immersed myself in what I called "all things Cambodian"—the history, art, dance, music, food, political situation, current events, research, and literature. I learned to enunciate some common phrases of greeting. At some point during my studies, I ventured to Angkor Wat alone, and I would like to return again someday. I had wanted to visit Tuol Sleng, but for various reasons, that was out of my reach at the time.

It took nearly 6 months of volunteering every weekend, and sometimes on special occasions, and driving the 90-mile round trip before I was finally accepted and recognized as a reliable volunteer. The community liaison had finally provided a name and put in me touch with another community member who could arrange in-person interviews and serve reliably as interpreter for the duration of my study.

The person who served as my interpreter was also valuable in locating, contacting, and arranging appointments and personal interviews. Over the next 4 to 5 months, we traveled to visit where the willing interviewees preferred to meet—their homes, businesses, temples, or the social services agency.

Unexpected and unknown to me beforehand, at one of the community celebrations, I was awarded "Volunteer of the Year." This was a great honor, and I still have the commemorative plaque.

This was my personal experience in gaining entre and establishing a level of trust with a community of people who had suffered much, yet remained hopeful for future generations.

Author: O. Catolico, 2023

Exemplar 2: Seeking Cultural Knowledge Through an Interpreter

An exemplar is an actual experience, lived, witnessed, or observed, used to illustrate or model those ideas, actions, or concepts expressed in the chapter. Note that aliases are used here in place of actual names to protect identities.

I was thrilled at the prospect of having an interpreter to be my guide in interviewing resettled Cambodian women, many of whom were older. The trusted community liaison at the social services agency referred me to Mr. Leung. Mr. Leung was an employee of the social services agency. He would schedule interview appointments ahead of time, and we negotiated and agreed upon monetary compensation for his time. I felt this was only fair, as he would be unavailable for other personal and professional commitments while serving as my interpreter. Mr. Leung was a certified medical interpreter who had previously worked in this capacity at a hospital in Washington State.

This particular interview took place in a private room of the local Buddhist temple. After prayer services and lunch, Mrs. Ban, a widow, agreed to be interviewed. The three of us sat on the floor on a bamboo mat. I faced Mrs. Ban and addressed my questions to her, with Mr. Leung sitting to the side nearby. We formed a little triangle.

At the beginning of the interview, I thanked Mrs. Ban for agreeing to spend time with me and explained the purpose of my interview—namely, to learn about how she views health and illness, and what she does to stay well. Since this was part of a research study, I obtained approval through my university's institutional review board to proceed with the study. Therefore, it was important before asking any questions to obtain her informed consent.

A hard copy of the informed consent was presented to her in English, and it was back translated into Khmer (the Cambodian language). I proceeded to explain to her in English that it is required of me to request her permission before proceeding to interview her. Mr. Leung aptly explained the same in Khmer. She took a moment to slowly and carefully read through the Khmer version of the consent form and replied "Yes, it is okay for you to ask me questions." She signed her own name at the bottom of the form.

I learned that Mrs. Ban was a survivor of "Pol Pot times" (1976–1979; Pol Pot was dictator during this time). She experienced atrocities under the Khmer Rouge (communist party). Her very signature on the consent form is significant for historical reasons and for her own lived experiences under the Khmer Rouge. During Pol Pot times people were forced to sign confessions and were executed. I was prepared in the event she might have chosen not to sign or to give her verbal consent.

Mrs. Ban related that she now lives with her adult daughter. She shared that she recently had gastric surgery and lifted her blouse slightly to show a well-healed epigastric scar. She indicates she has had "stomach problems" since Pol Pot times. I then asked simple follow-up questions, one at a time, through Mr. Leung about what led her to the hospital, what the hospitalization experience was like for her, and what she is doing now to stay well. A lengthy conversational exchange lasting nearly 10 minutes ensued between Mr. Leung and Mrs. Ban, without any return interpretation from Mr. Leung to me. During a brief pause, as Mr. Leung inhaled a breath before speaking again, I inserted, "What is happening? Will you please tell me what Mrs. Ban is saying?" To this Mr. Leung tersely replied, "She says she has no problems now." Although slightly flustered at the brevity of this reply, I managed to keep my composure and politely asked Mr. Leung to repeat the conversation I just witnessed, verbatim. He obliged and proceeded to explain that Mrs. Ban went to an American doctor and was sent away without any medication. She was upset at not having received any medication, but her adult daughter explained that an operation was needed to treat her effectively.

The most important thing that upset Mrs. Ban during her hospitalization was not the procedure or the postoperative pain, but the fact that she was not allowed to have or chew her betel seeds while hospitalized. She is glad now that she is out of the hospital and can chew her betel seeds whenever she wishes. The interview continued and lasted for about one hour, with Mr. Leung turning to me and providing an interpretative response after each question I asked of Mrs. Ban.

Mr. Leung and I took our leave of Mrs. Ban. During our post-interview debriefing, I explained that the details in the interviews I will be conducting are vitally important for the work I am doing. To this, Mr. Leung thoughtfully paused, and stated, "Oh ... ahh ... I see now. When I was the interpreter for the doctors in Washington, they did not want the details. They wanted short answers only. So I thought I should give you the same ... a short answer to what you want to know."

Having a clearer expectation of both of our roles, Mr. Leung was most valuable in facilitating entre to this community and in providing me with an emic perspective of Cambodian culture. He, too, was imprisoned and suffered starvation under the Khmer Rouge, as many did.

On some days we started out in the morning, stopped for lunch at a local Cambodian restaurant (owned and run by one of the interviewees), and proceeded with our task into late afternoon. My interview questions were not only answered with meaningful interpretation, but I had the privilege of seeing and meeting people who pushed beyond their past as they established their own businesses, reconnected with kin after years of separation, and helped build secure futures for their children by supporting them through college. "Hope" is the word that comes to mind.

Author: O. Catolico, 2023

References

Berlin, E. A., & Fowkes, W. C. (1983). A teaching framework for cross-cultural health care: Application in family practice. *The Western Journal of Medicine, 139*(6), 934–938.

Brislin, R. W. (1970). Back-translation for cross-cultural research. *Journal of Cross-Cultural Psychology, 1*(3), 185–216. https://doi.org/10.1177/135910457000100301

Centers for Disease Control and Prevention (CDC). (n.d.). *What is health literacy.* Retrieved June 30, 2023 from https://www.cdc.gov/healthliteracy/learn/index.html#print

Kleinman, A., & Benson, P. (2006, October). Anthropology in the clinic: The problem with cultural competency and how to fix it. *PLOS Medicine, 3*(10), Article e294. https://doi.org/10.1371/journal.pmed.0030294

Leininger, M. M. (2006). Culture care diversity and universality theory and evolution of the ethnonursing method. In M. M. Leininger & M. R. McFarland (Eds.), *Culture care diversity and universality: A worldwide nursing theory* (2nd ed., pp. 1–41). Jones & Bartlett.

Leininger, M.M. & McFarland, M.R. (2006). *Culture care diversity and universality: A worldwide nursing theory* (2nd ed.,). Jones & Bartlett.

Merriam-Webster Online Dictionary. *Worldview.* Retrieved on May 23, 2023, from https://www.merriam-webster.com/dictionary/worldview

National Association of Independent Schools (NAIS). (2018, June 22). *Kimberlé Crenshaw: Intersectionality: What is intersectionality* (1:54)[Video]. YouTube. https://www.youtube.com/watch?v=ViDtnfQ9FHc&t=57s

United States Department of Health and Human Services (USDHHS). (2021, May). *HIPAA for professionals.* Retrieved July 1, 2023, from https://www.hhs.gov/hipaa/for-professionals/index.html

Selected Bibliography

Bello, B. G., & Mancini, L. (2016). Talking about intersectionality: Interview with interview with Kimberlé W. Crenshaw. *Sociologia del Diritto, 2*, pp. 11–21. https://doi.org/10.3280/SD2016-002002

Catolico, O. (2015; 2021; 2023). Cultural perspectives: Cambodians. In *Lippincott advisor cultural perspectives*. [Computer software]. Lippincott. https://www.wolterskluwer.com/en/solutions/lippincott-solutions/lippincott-advisor

Catolico, O. (2022; 2024). Cultural perspectives: Veterans. In *Lippincott advisor cultural perspectives*. [Computer software]. Lippincott. https://www.wolterskluwer.com/en/solutions/lippincott-solutions/lippincott-advisor

Graham, E. A., & Chitnarong, J. (1997). Ethnographic study among Seattle Cambodians: Wind illness. *Ethnomed.* https://ethnomed.org/resource/ethnographic-study-among-seattle-cambodians-wind-illness/#

Hinton, D., Um, K., & Ba, P. (2001a). *Kyol Goeu* ("wind overload") part I: A cultural syndrome of orthostatic panic among Khmer refugees. *Transcultural Psychiatry, 38*(4), 403–432. https://doi.org/10.1177/136346150103800401

Hinton, D., Um, K., & Ba, P. (2001b). *Kyol Goeu* ("wind overload') part II: Prevalence, characteristics, and mechanisms of *Kyol Goeu* and near-*Kyol Goeu* episodes of Khmer patients attending a psychiatric clinic. *Transcultural Psychiatry, 38*(4), 433–460. https://doi.org/10.1177/136346150103800402

Kleinman, A., & Benson, P. (2006). Culture, moral experience, and medicine. *The Mount Sinai Journal of Medicine, 73*(6), 834–839.

Kleinman, A., Eisenberg, L., & Good, B. (2006). Culture, illness and care: Clinical lessons from anthropologic and cross-cultural research. *Focus: The Journal of Lifelong Learning in Psychiatry, 4*(1), 140–149.

Luna, L. J. (2002). Arab Muslims and culture care. In M. M. Leininger & M. R. McFarland (Eds.), *Transcultural nursing: Concepts, theories, research and practice* (3rd ed., pp. 301–311). McGraw Hill.

Morales, D. X., Beltran, T. F., & Morales, A. S. (2022). Gender, socioeconomic status, and COVID-19 vaccine hesitancy in the U.S.: An intersectionality approach. *Sociology of Health and Illness, 44*, 953–971. https://doi.org/10.1111/1467-9566.13474

Papke, R. L., Hatsukami, D. K., & Herzog, T. A. (2020). Betel quid, health, and addiction. *Substance Use & Misuse, 55*(9), 1528–1532. https://doi.org/10.1080/10826084.2019.1666147

Purnell, L. D. (2014). People of Arab heritage. In L. D. Purnell (Ed.), *Guide to culturally competent health care* (3rd ed., pp.101–117). F.A. Davis.

Roes, M., Uribe, F. L., Peters-Nehrenheim, V., Sits, C., Johannessen, A., Charlesworth, G., Parveen, S., Mueller, N., Jones, C. H., Thyrian, R., Monsees, J., & Tezcan-Guntekin, H. (2022). Intersectionality and its relevance for research in dementia care of people with a migration background. *Zeitchrift fur Gerontologie und Geriatrie, 55*, 287–291. https://doi.org/10.1007/s00391-022-02058-y

Santana, S., Brach, C., Harris, L., Ochiiai, E., Blakey, C., Bevington, F., Kleinman, D., & Pronk, N. (2021). Updating health literacy for Healthy People 2030: Defining its importance for a new decade in public health. *Journal of Public Health Management and Practice, 27*(6), Supplement. https://doi.org/10.1097/PHH0000000000001324

Stokes, C., Pino, J. A., Hagan, D. W., Torres, G. E., Phelps, E. A., Horenstein, N. A., & Papke, R. L. (2022). Betel quid: New insights into an ancient addiction. *Addiction biology, 27*(5), e13223. https://doi.org/10.1111/adb.13223

Van Herk, K. A., Smith, D., & Andrew, C. (2010). Examining our privileges and oppressions: Incorporating an intersectionality paradigm into nursing. *Nursing Inquiry, 18*(1), 29–39.

Wetzel, L. (1995). Cambodian cultural profile. *Ethnomed.* https://ethnomed.org/culture/cambodian/#

Websites

Transcultural Nursing Society https://tcns.org/theoriesandmodels/

United States Department of Health and Human Services Think Cultural Health:

National Culturally and Linguistically Appropriate Services Standards (CLAS) https://thinkculturalhealth.hhs.gov/clas/standards

Tracking CLAS https://thinkculturalhealth.hhs.gov/clas/clas-tracking-map

CLAS Behavioral Health Guide: Class Guide, Report, and Toolkit

https://minorityhealth.hhs.gov/clas-behavioral-health-implementation-guide

Culturally competent nursing care—A cornerstone of caring https://thinkculturalhealth.hhs.gov/education/nurses

Cultural Competency Program for Disaster Preparedness and Crisis Response https://thinkculturalhealth.hhs.gov/education/disaster-personnel

National CLAS Standards https://thinkculturalhealth.hhs.gov/clas/standards?utm_medium=email&utm_source=govdelivery

National CLAS Standards (English) https://thinkculturalhealth.hhs.gov/assets/pdfs/Enhanced NationalCLASStandards.pdf

How-to Guides https://thinkculturalhealth.hhs.gov/resources/library

Think Cultural Health Resource Library https://thinkculturalhealth.hhs.gov/resources/library

U.S. Department of Health and Human Services: Office of Minority Health https://www.minorityhealth.hhs.gov/

Webinars

Barksdale, C. (2015). *The context of CLAS in mental health* [Webinar]. U.S. Department of Health and Human Services. https://thinkculturalhealth.hhs.gov/resources/presentations/10/the-context-of-clas-in-mental-health-the-national-clas-standards

Graves, D. (2014). *The national CLAS standards, health literacy, and communication* [Webinar]. U.S. Department of Health and Human Services. https://thinkculturalhealth.hhs.gov/resources/presentations/8/the-national-clas-standards-health-literacy-and-communication

Graves, D. (2015). *Exploring culture in CLAS sexual orientation and gender identity* [Webinar]. U.S. Department of Health and Human Services. https://thinkculturalhealth.hhs.gov/resources/presentations/5/exploring-culture-in-clas-sexual-orientation-and-gender-identity

Graves, D. (2015). *Exploring culture in CLAS: Religion and spirituality* [Webinar]. U.S. Department of Health and Human Services. https://thinkculturalhealth.hhs.gov/resources/presentations/6/exploring-culture-in-clas-religion-and-spirituality

Graves, D., Tenorio, E., & Neumann, G. (2014). *The national standards for culturally and linguistically appropriate services in health and healthcare: A tool for tribal communities* [Webinar]. U.S. Department of Health and Human Services. https://thinkculturalhealth.hhs.gov/resources/presentations/14/the-national-standards-for-culturally-and-linguistically-appropriate-services-in-health

Webinar Presentation

Advancing behavioral health equity: National CLAS standards in action webinar (1:01:03) [Webinar]. U.S. Department of Health and Human Services, Office of Minority Health (2021, November 16) https://www.youtube.com/watch?v=UlmTDG87Fs

Videos: Transcultural Nursing Theory: Madeleine Leininger

Home Care of Rochester. (2008). *Dr. Madeleine Leininger interview, part 1* (12:02) [Video]. YouTube. https://www.youtube.com/watch?v=a4GTo_uthZQ

Home Care of Rochester. (2008). *Dr. Madeleine Leininger interview, part 2* (13:22) [Video]. YouTube. https://www.youtube.com/watch?v=6xchWCgeMM4

Ethnomed

Miyagawa, L. A. (2020). Practicing cultural humility when serving immigrant and refugee communities. *Ethnomed*. https://ethnomed.org/resource/practicing-cultural-humility-when-serving-immigrant-and-refugee-communities/#

Cultural brokering and advocacy-interpreting for patients with emotional trauma. (2016). *Ethnomed*. https://ethnomed.org/resource/cultural-brokering-advocacy-interpreting-for-patients-with-emotional-trauma/#

Ethnomed UW. (2019). Interpreting Pearls: Interpreting for Patients with Emotional Trauma Scenario 1 [Video]. YouTube. https://www.youtube.com/watch?v=bvrU30iCsXQ (2:02)

Ethnomed UW. (2019). Interpreting Emotional Trauma Scenario 1 Discussion (2:06) [Video]. YouTube. https://www.youtube.com/watch?v=HdFpedU_aZc

Ethnomed UW. (2019). Interpreting Pearls: Interpreting for Patients with Emotional Trauma Scenario 2 (3:02) [Video]. YouTube. https://www.youtube.com/watch?v=JpJOpzexysA

Ethnomed UW. (2019). Interpreting Emotional Trauma Scenario 2 Discussion (2:37) [Video]. YouTube. https://www.youtube.com/watch?v=an3izX4_vIg

Ethnomed UW. (2019). Interpreting Pearls: Interpreting for Patients with Emotional Trauma Scenario 3 (4:11) [Video]. YouTube. https://www.youtube.com/watch?v=k2_uGeEQAXk

Ethnomed UW. (2019). Interpreting Emotional Trauma Scenario 3 Discussion (1:37) [Video]. YouTube. https://www.youtube.com/watch?v=uvbHdzG40P4

Documentaries by Vivian Chavez

Chavez, V. (2012). Cultural Humility: People, Principles, and Practices—Part I of 4 (7:12) [Video]. YouTube.   https://www.youtube.com/watch?v=_Mbu8bvKb_U

Chavez, V. (2012). Cultural Humility: History, Poetry, Power and Privilege—Part 2 of 4 (8:58) [Video]. YouTube. https://www.youtube.com/watch?v=5a2X3Q4cUE0

Chavez, V. (2012). Cultural Humility in Community Based Participatory Research & Education, Part 3 of 4 (9:50) [Video]. YouTube. https://www.youtube.com/watch?v=9cEXqNDOHqM

Chavez, V. (2012). Cultural Humility—Closing Reflections, Part 4 of 4 (3:24) [Video]. YouTube. https://www.youtube.com/watch?v=HzEsuY2x2Ww

Chavez, V. (2012). Cultural Humility (complete) (29:28) [Video]. YouTube. https://www.youtube.com/watch?v=SaSHLbS1V4w

Intersectionality

Syracuse University Libraries. (n.d.). *FYS 101: Intersectional self.* https://researchguides.library.syr.edu/fys101/intersectionality

Anderson, K. (2017). *Kimberlé Crenshaw at Ted + animation* (5:57) [Video]. YouTube. https://www.youtube.com/watch?v=JRci2V8PxW4

Sociological Studies Sheffield. (2020). *Intersectionality and health explained* (3"35') [Video]. YouTube. https://www.youtube.com/watch?v=rwqnC1fy_zc

Medical Interpreters

National Board of Certification for Medical Interpreters https://www.certifiedmedicalinterpreters.org/

National Board of Certification for Medical Interpreters Registry https://www.certifiedmedical interpreters.org/search-cmi-registry

Certification Commission for Healthcare Interpreters https://cchicertification.org/

National Certified Interpreter Registry https://cchi.learningbuilder.com/Search/Public/MemberRole/Registry

TED Talks

Moseley, J. (2017). *Cultural humility: It makes all the difference* (16:49) [Video]. YouTube. https://www.ted.com/talks/juliana_mosley_ph_d_cultural_humility

Valles, S. (2018). *A culture of humility for a culture of health* (11:29) [Video]. YouTube. https://www.ted.com/talks/sean_valles_a_culture_of_humility_for_a_culture_of_health

Miscellaneous

Maben, A. (1997). *Dancing for the gods: Cambodia classical dance: Heritage of the ancient Khmer ancestors* (Documentary, 1997) [Video]. YouTube. https://www.youtube.com/watch?v=JkpXEPfxql0&t=293s

Image Credits

IMG 4.1: Copyright © 2021 Depositphotos/zurijeta.

Fig. 4.2: Adapted from Marilyn R. McFarland and Hiba B. Wehbe-Alamah, Leininger's Culture Care Diversity and Universality. Copyright © 2015 by Jones and Bartlett Learning.

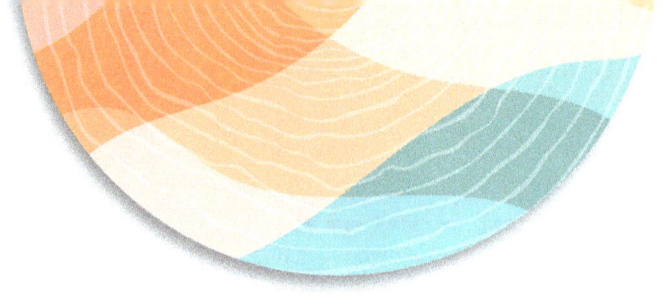

HEALTH DISPARITIES AND OLDER ADULTS

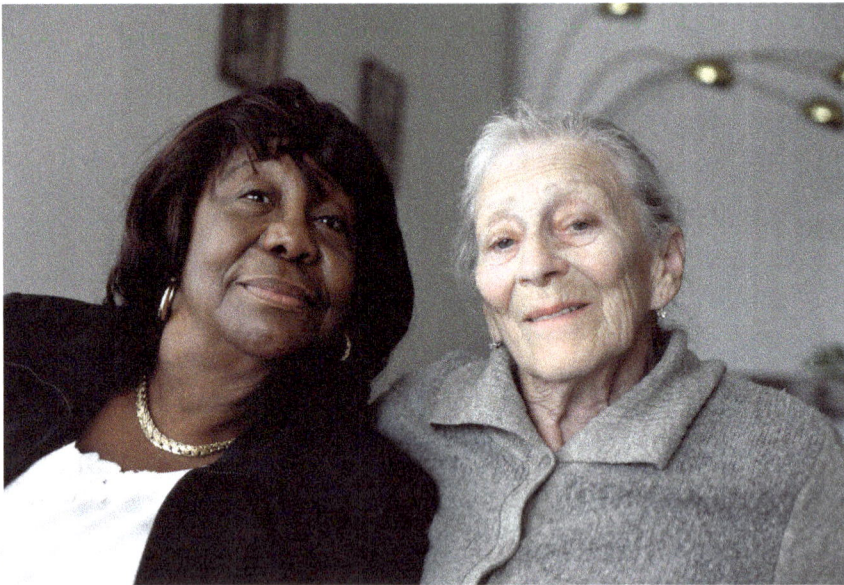

Image 5.1

Overview

The previous chapter provided the groundwork for exploring health disparities. An open discussion of health care disparities must also include concepts and discussions of diversity, equity, and inclusion. Health disparities continue to exist among marginalized groups of older adults. This chapter explores prevalent and ongoing systemic issues that contribute to disparities and inequities, particularly among ethnically diverse groups. The information in this chapter is intended to engage the reader in actively addressing health care inequities and disparities within their own professional practice, workplace, and communities.

Outcomes

The learner:

1. Defines key terms

   A. Disparities

   B. Diversity inclusion

   C. Equity

   D. Implicit bias

   E. Inclusion

   F. Intersectionality

   G. Marginalization

   H. Vulnerability

2. Examines current data and trends about health care disparities and health outcomes

3. Utilizes knowledge of aging, culture, and health care systems in understanding how these influence access and utilization of care

4. Explores power structures and how these influence health care experiences of ethnically diverse older adults

5. Identifies ways to skillfully advocate for and support improved health care for marginalized communities and individuals

Health Care Disparities

Health care disparities are differences in access to or availability of facilities and health services and variation in disease rates, their occurrence, and disabilities between groups defined by socioeconomic characteristics such as age, ethnicity, economic resources, gender, or geography.

Factors contributing to health care disparities are multifaceted and complex. The existence of health care disparities and their alleviation requires that equity and inclusion are integrated into cross-cutting and achievable goals for older adults regardless of age, health status, abilities, gender and orientation, socioeconomic status, and location.

At a most fundamental level, older persons need readily available and affordable access to care and resources to support personal health and well-being in the presence of changing health status and functional abilities. Persons in rural communities may face special challenges in access to quality care for a number of reasons: (a) scarcity of health care professionals committed to a stable practice in rural areas, (b) travel distance and location of the nearest health care facility, and (c) the level and continuum of services provided by the nearest health care facility. While the COVID-19 pandemic also brought about innovations in health care through technology (telehealth care, patient–health care provider videoconferencing), disparities are evident here as well. There are issues with eHealth literacy among older adults, along with issues of personal access and utilization of technology (Huang et al., 2023; Cox, 2020; Jutai & Tuazon, 2022).

Beyond self-care and family and relatives, who often provide immediate sources of aid and help, medical facilities and effective health-oriented programs in local communities and neighborhoods are vital for older adult populations to thrive. Such facilities and programs must have a stable, highly qualified cadre of professionals who collaboratively and consistently provide excellent care. Foundational to this community health care infrastructure is a culture of inclusion. For the purposes of this chapter, a culture of inclusion is that which embraces diversity and mutual respect for differences and consistently provides high quality, seamless, person-centered care and a continuum of services to older adults. Communities and health care infrastructures that embrace a culture of inclusion are also self-reflective in examining and improving on systemic factors, processes, and policies that bar inclusion. The most comprehensive level, beyond the individual and community-based health care infrastructure, is that of governments and nations, who have responsibility and accountability to their citizens (see Figure 5.1).

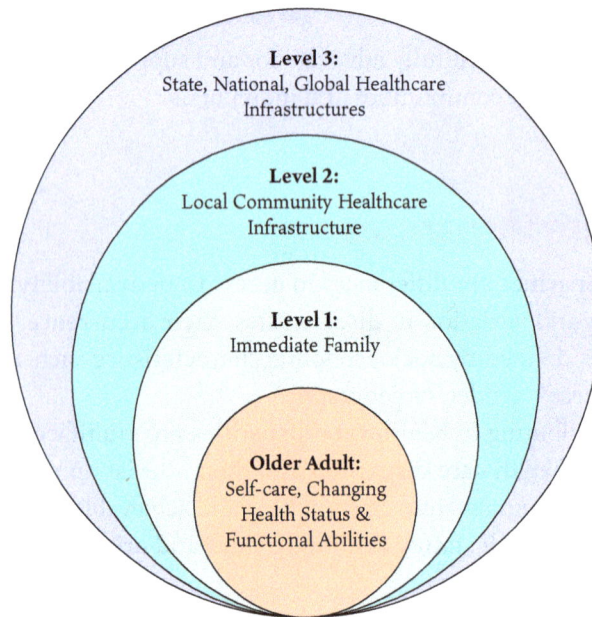

FIGURE 5.1   Levels of Inter-Related Health Care Support Systems for Older Adults

An additional factor to consider in alleviating disparities is that of implicit bias(es) in health care providers. Implicit bias comprises automatic and unintentional attitudes that affect decisions, behaviors, and actions of the health care provider. Ultimately, implicit bias influences care interactions, delivery, and patient outcomes. The concept of intersectionality also warrants discussion as it relates to health care disparities. Intersectionality is the interconnectedness of social categories, such as race, class, and gender, that create interdependent systems of discrimination or privilege and their relationship to power. Intersectionality is a lens to understand how categorizations may further exacerbate health care disparities, poor access to care, and poor outcomes. For example, Farrell et al. (2022) identify the intersection of ageism and racism in health care as a double disadvantage. Intersectionality is not limited to race, class, or gender, but extends also to social determinants of health. Unjust harm occurs at multiple levels of interaction among individuals and within and across health care institutions.

Marginalization is the process of placing people at the periphery of society based on their identity, associations, experiences, and environments (Hall et al., 1994), which contributes to inequities, barriers to care, and exclusion from society (Baah et al., 2018). Vulnerable populations experience unjust harm, marginalization, and stigma. Unsheltered persons, under-resourced and underserved minority communities, and communities of color, gender-diverse and neurodiverse persons, and persons who use illicit substances all experience health care disparities. The juxtaposition of multiple elements, such as intersectionality, marginalization, and systems issues and processes, perpetuate disparities.

When considered altogether, implicit bias, intersectionality, marginalization, and vulnerability place extreme burdens on older adults, who experience changes in health, functional abilities, personal losses, and diminished resources.

Social Determinants of Health and Health Disparities

The interaction of biological processes that occur in aging and social determinants of health may place the older adult at increased risk of poorer health. The U.S. Department of Health and Human Services for several years now has identified measurable target health goals for persons across the life cycle. There are identified targets for older adults. Worldwide, the World Health Organization (WHO) and the United Nations have identified Sustainable Development Goals, all of which are health-related and have an impact on the health and well-being of older adults. The extents to which SDGs are met are tracked by world region.

While governments at the local, state, and global levels disseminate reports and information about the health-related status of its citizens, health care systems and infrastructure are often fragmented. They may be beset by multiple factors, which may include issues with program development, monitoring and systematic evaluation, funding, staffing, leadership and management, specialized and/or conflicts of

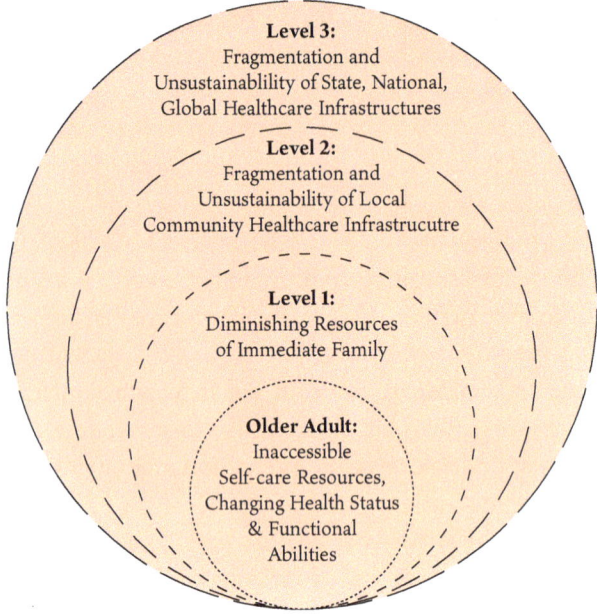

FIGURE 5.2　Consequences of Fragmented Systems of Care on the Older Adult

interests. Fractured programs at all levels ultimately impact health and increase a widening disparity gap contributing to marginalization and exclusion of vulnerable populations (see Figure 5.2).

Figure 5.2 illustrates levels of fragmentation with broken lines among the concentric circles. Those most affected are individuals and families. The widening distances between concentric circles as shown in Figure 5.2 illustrate the gaps that exist between enacted policies and processes at the state, national, and global levels, as well as the unrealized implementation and benefit to individuals and families.

Health Disparities and Ethical Treatment

Access to scientific advancements and effective treatments are also a determinant of health. The Agency for Healthcare Research and Quality submits to the U.S. Congress an annual report, National Healthcare Qualities and Disparities Report, to answer the question of *"How successfully does the nation ensure that people actually benefit from the scientific advancements and effective treatments available today?"* This question has particular relevance to older adult populations in the U.S.

Older adults, who are underrepresented, and persons of color are often excluded from participation in clinical trials. In addition, historically, past events have left their indelible marks on human experimental trials for the sake of science. One only needs to look back at the experiments of World War II and the syphilis study at Tuskegee to grasp the impact of history on present-day participation in clinical trials. On the one hand, pervasive mistrust may have an intergenerational impact affecting participation decisions, and on the other, past events have led to the passage of federal legislation, directives, and ethical codes governing scientific research on humans. The Nuremberg Code, the Declaration of Helsinki, and the Belmont Report are the foundations of informed consent for the protection of human subjects.

Effective and compassionate care for older adults also requires ethical reflection and practice on the part of the health care provider:

- Have current, accurate, and evidence-based information about all treatment options and interventions been provided to the older adult individual seeking care?

- Is this information provided in the preferred language of the older adult, or in other formats that are readily understood?

- If interpreters are used, are they certified medical interpreters?

- Has the individual seeking care expressed a gender preference of the interpreter, and has this been respected?

- Has the health care provider evaluated their own qualifications, expertise, and experience in the judicious administration of an evidence-based treatment or intervention in prescribing it for the older adult?

- Have benefits and consequences of evidence-based treatment been explained to the individual seeking care in a manner that is easily understood?

- Have clear explanations been provided to the individual about their participation in the treatment or intervention and what this entails (i.e., learning to administer a medication or procedure, cost of treatment/medication/supplies, participation in meetings, survey/interview completion, follow-up monitoring such as return visits to the health care provider, lab work)?

- Are support services readily available and accessible to the older adult individual as needed (health education and skills for care, interprofessional health care team)?

- Is the individual provided an opportunity to consider and weigh their treatment options and alternatives without duress or redress?

- Does the individual have an opportunity to seek a second opinion or consultation?

Praxis as introduced in a previous chapter requires intentional reflection, introspection, and a critical consciousness informed by a professional code of ethics. Being cognizant of these questions above may foster equity in practice.

Health Care Disparities and Evolving Issues

There is an abundance of current evidence showing that older adult populations were most vulnerable to the COVID-19 pandemic. Information from the Centers for Disease Control (CDC) National Center for Health Statistics shows that 81% of COVID-19 deaths in 2020 (282,836) occurred among those aged 65 and older. COVID-19 was the third leading cause of death in this age group after heart disease and cancer. Deaths from COVID-19 were higher for men than women. The death rate from COVID-19 for women aged 65 and older was highest for American Indian/Alaskan Native women, followed by non-Hispanic Black and Hispanic women (CDC, 2022). The implications of this pandemic should be a call to action for prevention, preparation, and recovery against the potential spread of harmful microorganisms.

Climate and environmental change is yet another evolving issue that has implications for older adults, particularly older adults who live in communities that are under-resourced and underserved. Extreme weather patterns and natural disasters leave a wake of problems for individuals who are frail, or who have limited functional ability or chronic illness. Older adults may live in homes built under older housing standards and with hazardous materials that pose health risks and are less energy efficient. Communities proximal to industrial plants or sites previously utilized for such a purpose place individuals at an increased risk for exposure to hazardous by-products and waste released into the environment. Illness, side effects, and exacerbation of existing medical conditions are often borne by people living in these communities. Recovery and rehabilitation from disasters also poses a financial burden to older adults, who may be living on a fixed income. Consequently, relocation, either temporary or permanent, may not be a viable option. These same communities may experience the absence of advocacy on their behalf, or are bereft of legislative representation or political voice to enact change within their respective communities (Dawes et al., 2022).

Influence and Advocacy: Closing the Health Care Disparity Gap

The compounding issues surrounding health care disparity among older adults presented in this chapter are not insurmountable. Intentional and deliberate efforts within one's circle of influence, at any level, will serve to make a difference. At the most fundamental level, older adults possess the ability to learn new information and skills for health maintenance and self-care. It is incumbent upon the health care provider to identify preferences and barriers to learning and to integrate culturally appropriate modes of learning (see Figure 5.3).

Level 1:	Level 2:	Level 3:	Level 4:
Education, health literacy for informed decision making, skills, support services	Family/caregiver education, resources, and support services, skills	Sustainable, accessible, programs and healthcare care infrastructure at community levels	Local, national, global policies and systems for health equity

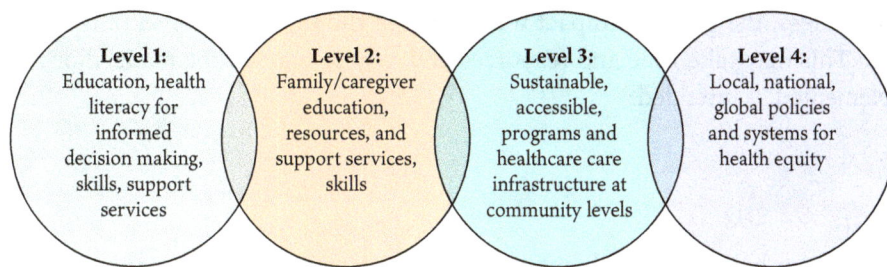

FIGURE 5.3 Effective Change, Advocacy, and Reflective Practice in One's Circle of Influence

Beyond the older individual's self-care are their families, who frequently take on the role of caregiver. Families also have informational and skills-based needs in their caregiving role. They, too, need support and respite services. Connecting the older adult and their family caregivers to community resources and support services is important in closing the disparity gap. This helps minimize the felt experiences of isolation, despair, and marginalization. As shown in Figure 5.3, communities should have health care infrastructure readily available and accessible to meet the needs of older adults and the families who support them. The health and well-being of individuals and families and the health and resilience of a community are interdependent. Therefore it is imperative that community-based health care-oriented programs and facilities maintain and sustain a high level of quality care.

There are several accrediting agencies that validate the quality of health care services. Accrediting agencies define and identify standards of care. Most importantly, the standards of care are measured, evaluated, and validated based on evidence. Among accrediting agencies are The Joint Commission (TJC), the Commission on Accreditation of Rehabilitation Facilities (CARF), and the Centers for Medicare and Medicaid Services (CMS). State agencies under the respective departments of public health, licensing, and certification also regulate and license health care facilities. Health care facilities also seek to improve care by collecting specific information from patients about their health care providers. One example is the Hospital Consumer Assessment of Healthcare Providers and Systems (HCAHPS). Facilities may also utilize other rigorous external standards to assure that health care providers employed by these facilities have the necessary education and maintain their expertise and qualifications. Certification of health care providers through nationally recognized professional associations is one way of achieving this.

An approach to help minimize health care disparity gaps at the broadest level of influence, the national or global levels, is providing input or feedback to legislative proposals that may have a wide impact. Having a voice on issues can be achieved through community action; joining community-oriented health care groups, professional organizations, or associations; and communicating with elected officials. Proposals at the country or global level may be well-intentioned to achieve change.

Nonetheless, the greatest impact will be felt at the individual level of the older adult. This may take time and resources and may or may not be realized or fully implemented as intended.

Chapter Summary

This chapter has introduced and reviewed key terms related to health care disparities. Health care disparities are influenced by Social Determinants of Health. Disparities exist at multiple levels of society—individual, group, community, and national or global. Fragmented health care infrastructure and services affect access to timely, quality care. Suggestions are offered about ways in which disparity can be addressed at multiple levels of society.

Glossary

Disparities: Health care disparities are differences in access to or availability of medical facilities and services and variation in rates of disease occurrence and disabilities between population groups defined by socioeconomic characteristics such as age, ethnicity, economic resources, or gender, and populations identified geographically (Agency for Healthcare Research and Quality, n.d.).

Diversity: Recognizing and valuing all the different characteristics that make one individual or group different from another, including not only race, ethnicity, and gender—the groups that most often come to mind when this term is used—but also age, national origin, religion, disability status, gender identity, sexual orientation, socioeconomic status, education, marital status, language, physical appearance, as well as different ideas, perspectives, and values (see Chapter 4).

Equity: Health equity is the attainment of the highest level of health for all people (USDHHS, n.d.). "Health equity is defined as the absence of unfair and avoidable or remediable differences in health among population groups defined socially, economically, demographically or geographically" (WHO, n.d.).

Implicit bias: Bias is prejudiced attitudes, behaviors, or actions against one person or group over another. *Implicit* bias is an automatic and unintentional bias affecting judgments, decisions, and behaviors (National Institutes of Health, n.d.).

Inclusion: Active, intentional, and ongoing engagement with diversity—in people, communities, agencies, institutions, organizations (intellectual, social, economic, cultural, geographical)—with which individuals connect in ways that increase one's awareness, knowledge, and cognitive and empathic understanding of the complex ways individuals interact within and change systems and institutions (Dominican University of California, n.d.).

Intersectionality: A framework for understanding the interconnectedness of social categorizations (such as race, class, gender) that create interdependent systems of discrimination and disadvantage, or privilege; social identities and its relationship to power (NAIS, 2018; Cho, Crenshaw, & McCall, 2013).

Marginalization: The process of placing people at the periphery of society based on their identity, associations, experiences, and environments (Hall et al., 1994), which contributes to structural and social inequities. Inherent in marginalization is power and dominance exerted over others, which creates physical, emotional, and psychological boundaries. Marginalization creates barriers, social exclusion, and vulnerabilities (Baah et al., 2018).

Vulnerability: Being exposed to or unprotected from health-damaging environments (Hall et al., 1994).

References

Agency for Healthcare Research & Quality. (n.d.). *Disparities*. Retrieved July 10, 2023, from https://www.ahrq.gov/topics/disparities.html

Baah, F. O., Teitelman, A. M. & Riegel, B. (2018). Marginalization: Conceptualizing patient vulnerabilities in the framework of social determinants of health—An integrative review. *Nursing Inquiry, 26*(1). https://doi.org/10.1111/nin.12268

Dawes, D. E., Donnell, M., Amador, C., Standifer, M., Valle, M., Houston, S., McKinney, T., & Dunlap, N. (2022). The political determinants of health and health equity in the aging population. *Generations Journal, 46*, 1–17

Cho, S., Crenshaw, K.W., & McCall, L. (2013). Toward a filed of intersectionality studies: Theory, applications, and Praxis. *Journal of Women in Culture and Society, 38*(4), 785-810

Dominican University of California. (n.d.). *Seven dimensions of fostering diversity, equity, & inclusion: A strategic plan for Dominican University of California, 2020–2025.* Retrieved July 10, 2023, from https://www.dominican.edu/sites/default/files/2021-03/DAG-7Dimensions-Feb2021-Final.pdf

Centers for Disease Control (CDC). (2022). Covid-19 mortality in adults aged 65 and over: United States, 2020. *National Center for Health Statistics Data Brief, 446.* https://www.cdc.gov/nchs/data/databriefs/db446.pdf

Cox, C. (2020). Older adults and Covid 19: Social justice, disparities, and social work practice. *Journal of Gerontological Social Work, 63*(6/7). https://doi:10.1080/01634372.2020.1808141

Farrell, T. W., Hung, W. W., Unroe, K. T., Brown, T. R., Furman, C. D., Jih, J., Karani, R., Mulhausen, P., Napoles, A. M., Nnodim, J. O., Upchurch, G., Whittaker, C. F., Lim, A., Lundebjerg, N. E., & Rhodes, R. L. (2022). Exploring the intersection of structural racism and ageism in healthcare. *Journal of the American Geriatrics Society, 70*(12). https://doi.org/10.1111/jgs.18105

Hall, J. M., Stevens, P. E., & Meleis, A. I. (1994). Marginalization: A guiding concept for valuing diversity in nursing knowledge development. *Advances in Nursing Science, 16*(4), 23–41.

Huang, Q. Y., Liu, L., Goodarzi, Z., & Watt, J. A. (2023). Diagnostic accuracy of eHealth literacy measurement tools in older adults: A systematic review. *BMC Geriatrics, 23*(181), 1–10. https://doi.org/10.1186/s12877-023-03899-x

Jutai, J. W., & Tuazon, J. R. (2022). The role of assistive technology in addressing social isolation, loneliness and health inequities among older adults during the COVID-19 pandemic. *Disability and Rehabilitation Assistive Technology, 17*(3), 248–259. https;//doi.org/10.1080/17483107.2021. 2021305

National Association of Independent Schools (NAIS). (2018, June 22). *Kimberlé Crenshaw: Intersectionality: What is intersectionality* (1:54)[Video]. YouTube. https://www.youtube.com/watch?v=ViDtnfQ9FHc&t=57

National Institutes of Health. (n.d.). *Implicit bias.* https://diversity.nih.gov/general-page/implicit-bias

United States Department of Health & Human Services (USDHHS). (n.d.). *Health equity in Healthy People 2030.* Office of Disease Prevention & Health Promotion. Retrieved July 10, 2023, from https://health.gov/healthypeople/priority-areas/health-equity-healthy-people-2030

World Health Organization (WHO). (n.d.). *Social determinants of health: Health equity.* Retrieved July 10, 2023, from https://www.who.int/health-topics/social-determinants-of-health#tab=tab_3

Selected Bibliography

Ackerman, L. S. & Chopik, W. J. (2021). Cross-cultural comparisons in implicit and explicit age bias. *Personality and Social Psychology Bulletin, 47*(6), 953–968. https://doi.org/10.1177/01461672 20950070

Agenor, M. (2020). Future directions for incorporating intersectionality into quantitative population health research. *American Journal of Public Health, 110*(6), 803–806. https://doi.org/10.2105/AJPH.2020.305610

American Association of Retired Persons (AARP). *Disaster Resilience Toolkit* https://www.aarp.org/content/dam/aarp/livable-communities/tool-kits-resources/2022/AARP%20Disaster%20Resilience%20Tool%20Kit-singles-060122-.pdf

Braveman, P. (2014). What are health disparities and health equity? We need to be clear. *Public Health Reports, 129*(5–8). https://doi.org/10.1177/00333549141291S203

Butterfield, P. G. (2002). Upstream reflections on environmental health. *Advances in Nursing Science, 25*(1), 32–49.

Boltz, M., BeLue, R., Resnick, B., Kuzmik, A., Galik, E., Jones, J. R., Arendacs, R., Sinvani, L., Mogle, J., & Galvin, J. E. (2021). Disparities in physical and psychological symptoms in hospitalized African American and White persons with dementia. *Journal of Aging and Health, 33*(5–6), 340–349. https://doi.org/10.1177/0898264320983210

Caskie, G. I. L., Patterson, S. L., & Voelkner, A. R. (2022). Health bias in clinical work with older adult clients: The relation with ageism and aging anxiety. *Clinical Gerontologist, 45*(2), 351–365. https://doi.org/10.1080/07317115.2021.2019863

Conner, K. O., Wiltshire, J., Garcia, E. C., Langland-Orban, B., Anderson, E., Carrion, I., Goodman, A., & Goodman, A. (2022). Racial and ethnic differences in cost-of-care conversations among older adults. *Journal of Communication in Healthcare, 15*(3), 178–188. https://doi.org/10.1080/17538068.2022.2072165

Cummings-Vaughn, L. (2023). Health disparities in long-term care for people living with dementia. *Generations Journal, 47*(1), 1–9.

Federal Emergency Management System (FEMA). *Making the Connection to Older Adults: Guide to Expanding Mitigation.* https://www.fema.gov/sites/default/files/documents/fema_mitigation-guide_older-adults.pdf

Ghasemi, E., Majdzadeh, R., Rajabi, F., Vedadhir, A., Negarandeh, R., Jamshidi, E., Takian, A., & Faraji, Z. (2021). Applying intersectionality in designing and implementing health interventions: A scoping review. *BMC Public Health, 21*(1407), 1–13. https://doi.org/10.1186/s12889-021-11449-6

Hall, J. M., & Carlson, K. (2016). Marginalization: A revisitation with integration of scholarship on globalization, intersectionality, privilege, microaggressions, and implicit biases. *Advances in Nursing Science, 39*(3), 200–215. https://doi.org/10.1097/ANS.0000000000000123

Henning-Smith, C. (2020). The unique impact of COVID-19 on older adults in rural areas. *Journal of Aging and Social Policy, 32*(4–5), 396–402. https://doi.org/10.1080/08959420.2020.1770036

Hill, J. D., De Forecrand, C., Cuthel, A. M., Adeyemi, O. J., Shallcross, A. J., & Grudzen, C. R. (2022). Emergency provider perspectives on facilitators and barriers to home and community services for older adults with serious life limiting illness: A qualitative study. *PLOS One, 17*(8), 1–11. https://doi.org/10.1371/journal.pone.0270961

Jain, B., Khatri, E., Stanford, F. C. (2021). Racial disparities in senior healthcare: System-level interventions. *Journal of the American Geriatrics Society, 70*, 1292–1296. https://doi.org/10.1111/jgs.7658

Lampe, N. M. (2022). Liminal lives in uncertain times: Health management during the COVID-19 pandemic among transgender and non-binary older adults. *Gerontology & Geriatric Medicine, 8*, 1–8. https://doi.org/10.1177/23337214221127753

Lesser, S., Zakharkin, S., Louie, C., Escobedo, M. R., Whyte, J., & Fulmer, T. (2021). Clinician knowledge and behaviors related to the 4Ms framework of age-friendly health systems. *Journal of the American Geriatrics Society, 70*, 789–800. https://doi.org/10.1111/jgs.17571

Lundebjerg, N. E., & Medina-Walpole, A. M. (2021). Future forward: AGS initiative addressing intersection of structural racism and ageism in health care. *Journal of the American Geriatrics Society, 69*, 892–895. https://doi.org/10.1111/jgs.17053

Moreno, O., Garcia-Rodriguez, I., Fuentes, L., Hernandez, C., Munoz, G., Fluellen, K., Hobgood, S., & Sargent, L. Non-Latinx healthcare provider's knowledge and awareness of Latinx geriatric clinical health needs. *Clinical Gerontologist, 46*(2), 168–179. https://doi.org/10.1080/07317115.2022.2065943

Naik, A. D. (2022). Measuring patient-centered care to improve hospital experiences of older adults. *Journal of the American Geriatrics Society, 70*, 3348–3351. https://doi.org/10.1111/jgs.18048

National Academies of Sciences, Engineering, and Medicine. (2017). *Communities in action: Pathways to health equity.* The National Academies Press. https://doi.org/10.17226/24624

Ornstein, K. A., Garrido, M. M., Bollens-Lund, E., Reckrey, J. J., Husain, M., Ferreira, K. B., Liu, S., Ankuda, C. K., Kelley, A. S., & Siu, A. L. (2020). The association between income and incident homebound status among older Medicare beneficiaries. *Journal of the American Geriatrics Society, 68*, 2594–2601. https://doi.org/10.1111/jgs.16715

Thomas, N. D., & Leon, R. (2021). Future directions of care management: Care management in a world of many cultures. *Generations Journal, 45*(1), 1–11.

Todt, K. (2023). Strategies to combat implicit bias in nursing: Take steps to protect patient and nurse well-being. *American Nurse Journal, 18*(7), 1–10.

United States Department of Health and Human Services (USDHHS). (2022). *Health equity and health disparities environmental scan: Final report.* Office of Disease Prevention and Health Promotion.

Zulquarnain, J., Maqsood, M. H., Amin, Z., & Nasir, K. (2022). Race and ethnicity and cardiometabolic risk profile: Disparities across income and health insurance in a national sample of U.S. adults. *Journal of Public Health Management and Practice, 28*, S91–S100. https://doi.org/10.1097/PHH.0000000000001441

Websites

Centers for Disease Control and Prevention: The U.S. Public Health Service Syphilis Study at Tuskegee https://www.cdc.gov/tuskegee/index.html; https://www.cdc.gov/tuskegee/timeline.htm

Climate Science https://climatescience.org/

Hospital Consumer Assessment of Healthcare Providers and Systems Survey (HCAHPS) https://www.hcahpsonline.org/

Survey Instruments https://www.hcahpsonline.org/en/survey-instruments/

Hospital Survey https://www.ahrq.gov/cahps/surveys-guidance/hospital/index.html

Patients' Perspective of Care Survey https://www.cms.gov/medicare/quality-initiatives-patient-assessment-instruments/hospitalqualityinits/hospitalhcahps

NASA Global Climate Change https://climatescience.org/

National Institute on Aging: Health Disparities https://www.nia.nih.gov/news/topics/health-disparities?page=0

The Joint Commission https://www.jointcommission.org/who-we-are/

United Nations Climate Action: What is Climate Change https://www.un.org/en/climatechange/what-is-climate-change

United States Department of Health and Human Services: The Belmont Report https://www.hhs.gov/ohrp/regulations-and-policy/belmont-report/index.html

United States Department of Health and Human Services Office of Research Integrity: The Nuremberg Code https://ori.hhs.gov/content/chapter-3-The-Protection-of-Human-Subjects-nuremberg-code-directives-human-experimentation

World Medical Association: Declaration of Helsinki https://www.wma.net/what-we-do/medical-ethics/declaration-of-helsinki/

Selected Videos

Crenshaw, K. (2016). *The urgency of intersectionality* (18 min 40 sec) [Video]. TED Women. https://www.ted.com/talks/kimberle_crenshaw_the_urgency_of_intersectionality?language=en

The Institute of Art and Ideas. (2021). *Kimberlé Crenshaw on intersectionality: The big idea* (5 min 14 sec) [Video]. YouTube. https://www.google.com/search?client=firefox-b-1-d&q=kimberle+crenshaw+video#fpstate=ive&vld=cid:d6fb2172,vid:-BnAW4NyOak

National Association of Independent Schools (NAIS). (2018). *Kimberlé Crenshaw: What is intersectionality?* (1 min 55 sec) [Video]. YouTube. https://www.youtube.com/watch?v=ViDtnfQ9FHc&t=57s

Thunberg, G. (2018). *School strike for climate change* (11 min 11 sec) [Video]. TEDx Stockholm. https://www.ted.com/talks/greta_thunberg_the_disarming_case_to_act_right_now_on_climate_change?language=en

Image Credits

IMG 5.1: Copyright © 2013 Depositphotos/logoboom.

MIGRATION AND AGING

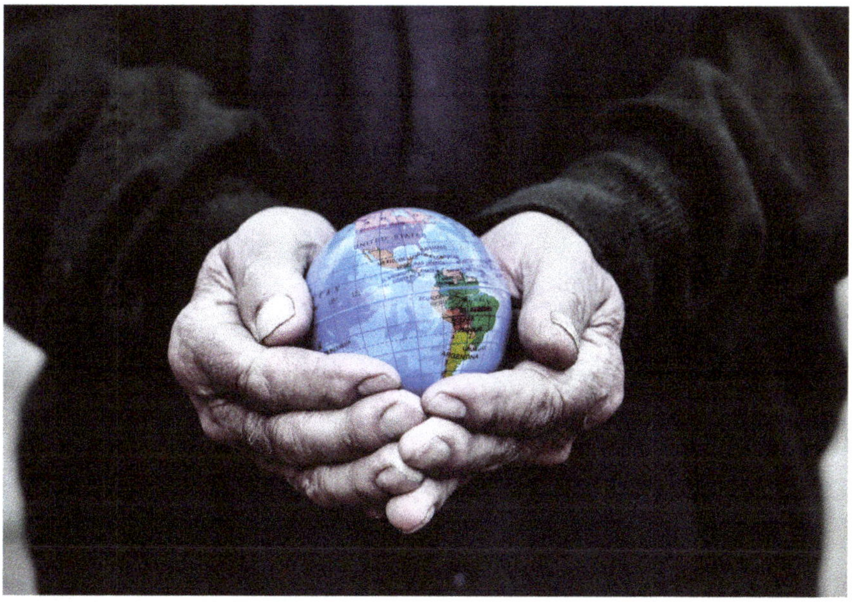

Image 6.1

Overview

Aging is a developing life event occurring globally. Family ties and socio-economic, environmental, and political factors influence where people age, whether by choice or not. Demographic shifts in the aging population occur as a result of migration. Subsequently, migration also influences the older adult's health and well-being. This chapter explores issues of migration and their health implications for the older adult.

Outcomes

The learner:

1. Defines key terms

   A. Displacement

   B. Immigration

   C. International migrant

   D. Migration

   E. Naturalization

   F. Refugee

   G. Relocation

   H. Resettlement

   I. Repatriation

2. Understands data trends and patterns related to older adult population shifts resulting from migration

3. Examines the dynamics and complex factors surrounding migration

4. Explores ethical issues related to health care of migrant populations of older adults

5. Explores systems and infrastructure issues that pose barriers to timely and effective health care for older adults

6. Articulates the immediate and long-term health consequences of delayed or absent care for older adult migrant populations

7. Demonstrates application of professional knowledge, interpersonal-intercultural communication skills, and characteristics in the process of eliciting vital health histories and health assessments

8. At the point of care, engages the older adult in decision-making and seeks timely and appropriate interventions to support or maintain health and well-being

Migration

Migration is the movement of people from one location to another. Definitions associated with migration and the context in which these terms are often used are listed in the glossary. This chapter focuses on health-related issues and outcomes brought about by migration instead of the legal-political ramifications. Movement of older adults from one place to another creates its own stresses. Although legal-political issues are sometimes intertwined with migration, the ability and capacity of people to maintain health is central to effectively managing and coping with change from one habitual residence to another (Figure 6.1).

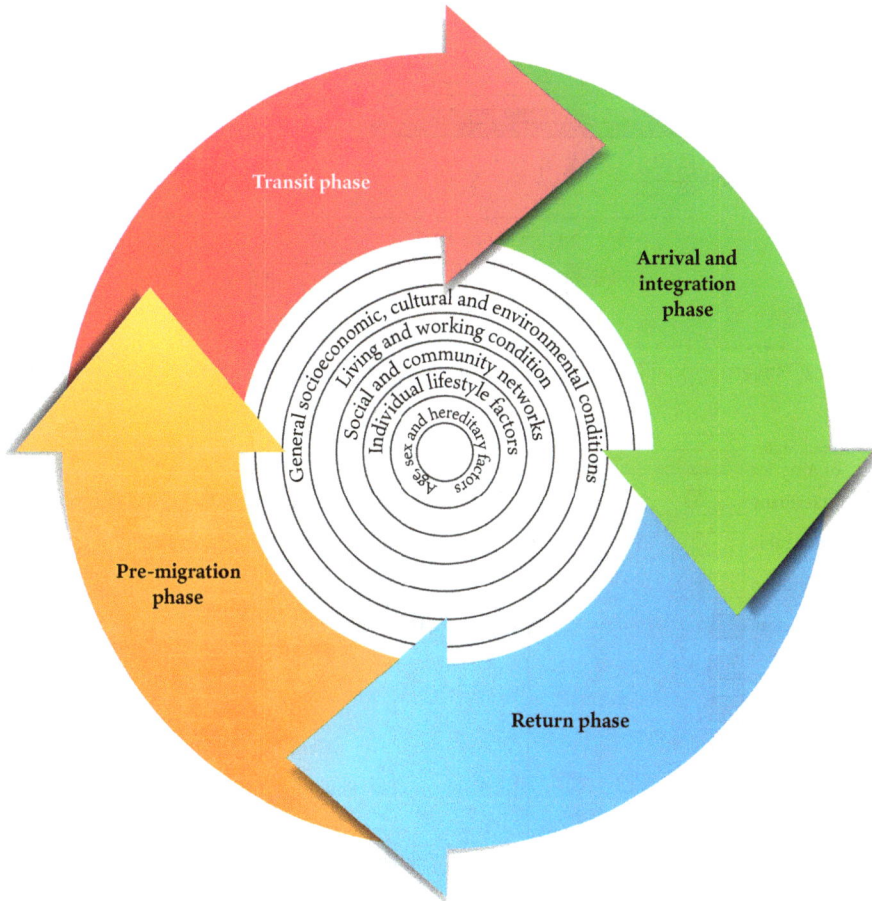

FIGURE 6.1 Determinants of Health and Phases of Migration

Migration Trends, Patterns, and Population Shifts

Migration may be short- or long-term, temporary, permanent, or indefinite. Migrational shifts occur across world regions. In 2020 there were 280.6 million global migrants, which represented nearly 4% of the world's population of 7.8 billion. Between 2010 and 2020, there were nearly 60 million people living outside their origin countries, owing largely to labor or family migration. This is a decrease compared to the 77.1 million international migrants noted in 1960. The percentage of the world's population comprising international migrants has risen steadily from 2.6% in 1960 to 3.2% in the previous decade, and to 3.6% in 2020 (Figure 6.2).

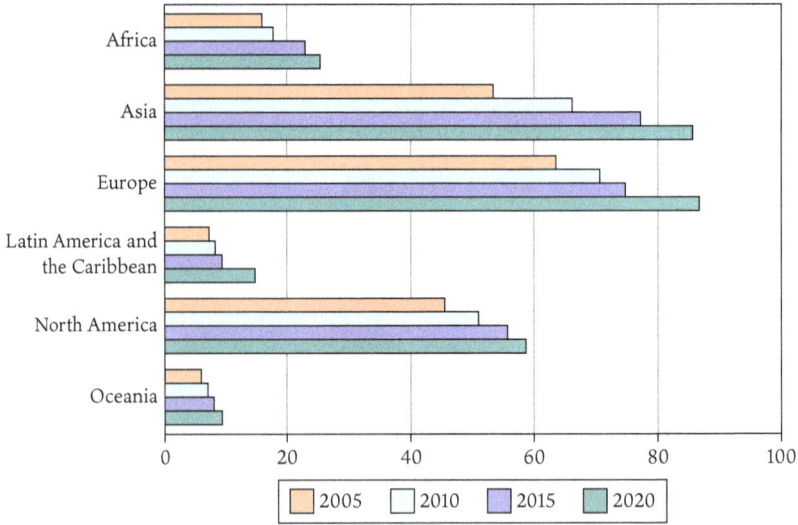

FIGURE 6.2 International Migrants by Major Region of Residence, 2005–2020 (millions)

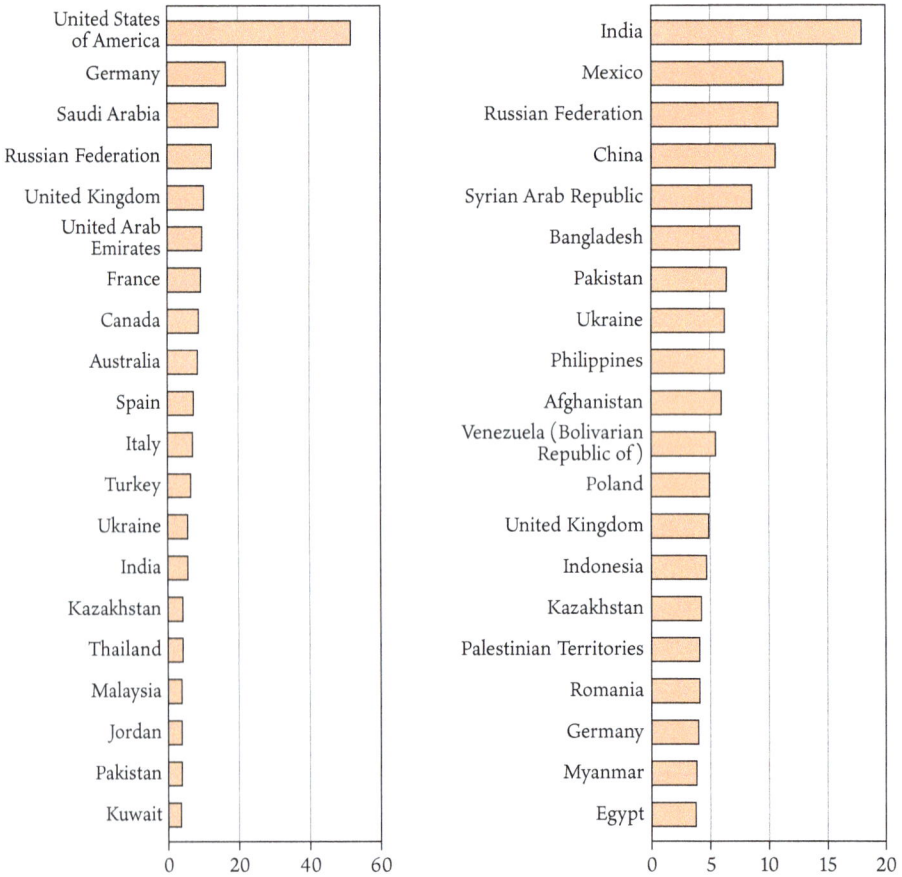

FIGURE 6.3 Top 20 Destinations (left) and Origins (right) of International Migrants in 2020 (millions)

Many migrants choose to go to high-income countries, such as the U.S. and Europe, for economic and social stability. Gulf countries also attract international migrants because of temporary worker programs (United Nations, n.d.; Table 6.1). The United States is the top destination for international migrants, followed by Germany, Saudi Arabia, the Russian Federation, the United Kingdom, and the United Arab Emirates (Figure 6.3). Although the U.S. is the top destination, the immigrant share of the total population in the U.S. is 15.3%, as compared to 88.1% in the United Arab Emirates (Migration Policy Institute, n.d.-b; Table 6.2; Figure 6.3).

TABLE 6.1 Destinations for International Migrants by Region, 2020

Destination	Number	Share of International Migrant Population (%)
Total International Migrant Population	**280,598,105**	**100%**
Europe and Northern America	145,414,863	52%
Northern Africa and Western Asia	49,767,746	18%
Sub-Saharan Africa	22,221,538	8%
Eastern and Southeastern Asia	19,591,106	7%
Central and Southern Asia	19,427,576	7%
Latin America and the Caribbean	14,794,623	5%
Australia and New Zealand	9,067,584	3%
Oceania (excluding Australia and New Zealand)	313,069	0%

Source: International migrant stock 2020 (United Nations, n.d.). https://www.un.org/development/desa/pd/content/international-migrant-stock

TABLE 6.2 Top 25 Destinations of International Migrants and Migrant Share of Total Populations

	Countries of Destination	Total Country Population	Migrant Share of Total Population (%)
1	United States of America	331,063,000	15.3%
2	Germany	83,784,000	18.8%
3	Saudi Arabia	34,814,000	38.6%
4	Russian Federation	145,934,000	8.3%
5	United Kingdom	67,886,000	13.8%
6	United Arab Emirates	9,890,000	88.1%
7	France	65,274,000	13.1%

continued

TABLE 6.2 *continued*

• •

8	Canada	37,742,000	21.3%
9	Australia	25,500,000	31.1%
10	Spain	46,755,000	14.6%
11	Italy	60,462,000	10.6%
12	Turkey	84,339,000	7.2%
13	Ukraine	43,734,000	11.4%
14	India	1,380,004,000	0.4%
15	Kazakhstan	18,777,000	19.9%
16	Thailand	69,800,000	5.2%
17	Malaysia	32,366,000	10.7%
18	Jordan	10,203,000	33.9%
19	Pakistan	220,892,000	1.5%
20	Kuwait	4,271,000	72.8%
21	China, Hong Kong Special Administrative Regions	7,497,000	39.5%
22	South Africa	59,309,000	4.8%
23	Iran Islamic Republic of	83,993,000	3.3%
24	Japan	126,476,000	2.2%
25	Cote d'Ivoire	26,378,000	9.7%

Sources: Top 25 destinations of international migrants (Migration Policy Institute, n.d.-b). https://www.migra-tionpolicy.org/programs/data-hub/charts/top-25-destinations-international-migrants
International Migrant Stock 2020 (United Nations, n.d., Destination: Table 1). www.un.org/development/desa/pd/content/international-migrant-stock

In the U.S., the population of persons who have migrated to the U.S. has slowed since 2015, which reflects the slowed growth of the U.S. population overall. Between 2014 and 2016, the immigrant population grew to 1.3 million. From 2017 to 2019, there were an additional 407,000 immigrant persons. From 2019 to 2021, additional immigrant persons numbered at 337,000 (Ward & Batalova, 2023). In 2022, there were about 46.2 million immigrants residing in the U.S., with few aged 65 years and older (Table 6.3). Older adults are less likely to migrate, and some may choose to return to their origin countries for retirement. Mortality is another factor accounting for the lower numbers of immigrants aged 65 years and older. In contrast, the native-born U.S. population aged 65 years and older are greater in number in 2022 as a result of the "baby boom," the increased numbers of people born post-World War II between 1946 and 1964 (Migration Policy Institute, n.d.-a).

TABLE 6.3 Age-Sex Distribution of Immigrant and U.S.-Born Populations 2022

Immigrants (2022)			U.S.-Born Population (2022)		
Age Group	Male	Female	Age Group	Male	Female
85+	312,000	585,200	85+	1,906,100	3,361,700
	34.8%	65.2%		36.1%	63.9%
	0.7%	1.3%		0.7%	1.2%
80–84	404,000	606,900	80–84	2,456,800	3,290,800
	40.0%	60.0%		42.7%	57.3%
	0.9%	1.3%		0.9%	1.1%
75–79	629,700	859,700	75–79	4,271,900	5,244,200
	42.3%	57.7%		44.9%	55.1%
	1.4%	1.7%		1.5%	1.8%
70–74	946,800	1,129,700	70–74	6,203,100	7,059,000
	45.6%	54.4%		46.8%	53.25%
	2.1%	2.4%		2.2%	2.5%
65–69	1,262,300	1,448,700	65–69	7,536,700	8,311,900
	46.6%	53.4%		47.6%	52.4%
	2.7%	3.1%		2.6%	2.9%
60–64	1,626,000	1,771,100	60–64	8,866,500	9,310,200
	47.9%	52.1%		48.8%	51.2%
	3.5%	3.8%		3.1%	3.2%
55–59	1,944,900	2,001,500	55–59	8,218,500	8,388,700
	49.3%	50.7%		49.5%	50.5%
	4.2%	4.3%		2.9%	2.9%
Data for ages 0–54 excluded			Data for ages 0–54 excluded		

Total Immigrant Population: 46,182,200   Total U.S. Born Population: 287,105,400

Immigrant Male:

🟦 Share immigrant population by age category

🟩 Share of total immigrant population

Immigrant Female:

🟨 Share immigrant population by age category

🟥 Share of total immigrant population

Source: IPUMS USA: Version 12.0 [dataset] (Ruggles et al., 2022). https://www.ipums.org/projects/ipums-usa/d010.v12.0

Aging Societies

Global population growth continues an upward climb, from 2.5 billion in 1950 to 8 billion in 2022. It is projected to grow to 9.7 billion in 2050. Globally, people 65 years of age and older exceed the population of children under age 5. This trend is notable in high- and upper-middle-income countries. The share of people over age 65 in high-income countries was historically high at 10% in 2022. This share is expected to increase to 29% by 2050. The ratio of working-age adults (20–64 years) to elderly (65 years and above) dipped from 7.1 in 1950 to 2.9 in 2022. This ratio is expected to further decrease to below 2.0 mid-century (World Bank, 2023). These trends and projections provide substance for social protection programs and effective policies. Upper-middle- and middle-income countries also have a declining work-age population (20–64 years). By mid-century, low-income countries are expected to experience population growth in which children under age 5 will exceed elderly persons (age 65 and older).

Migration and the Impact of COVID-19

Recent and comprehensive data about migration shifts in global regions are captured by the International Organization for Migration (IOM; https://www.iom.int/), the World Health Organization (WHO; https://www.who.int/), the United Nations (UN; https://www.un.org/en/), and the United Nations Refugee Agency, United Nations High Commissioner for Refugees (UNHCR; https://www.unhcr.org/).

Many governments worldwide imposed intercontinental, regional, and domestic travel restrictions during the COVID-19 pandemic. Stringent health mandates were also widely enforced with any travel. Although severe COVID restrictions have been retracted, the repercussions of the pandemic continue to impact people at many levels, even as recovery efforts have been underway. For example, the pandemic abruptly halted the lives of many who were dependent on migration to earn a living. People who migrated within country or across international borders for work were left in precarious situations. They were unable to return home or stranded in undesirable environments and lost employment and income. Thus, families left at home, including older adults and extended family, perhaps still are lacking financial resources for living. In countries where migrant persons were employed, the temporariness of their work situation and residence status further compounded their health status, as access to COVID vaccinations were delayed or unavailable.

The IOM *World Migration Report 2022* (2021) provides data on migration in global regions. Reported information may exclude entry bans related to visa restrictions, citizenship, and departure and exit restrictions, all of which severely limited mobility during the pandemic.

Africa

Intra-African travel restrictions were enacted in 2020, with health measures (i.e., quarantine and negative COVID tests). Health measures were in place in more than 80% of country-to-country corridors in the African region in 2021. Africa holds many displaced people, including refugees and asylum seekers, largely due to protracted conflict within the region. The origin countries of displaced persons include South Sudan, the Democratic Republic of the Congo, and Somalia. Uganda has hosted approximately 1.4 million displaced persons from surrounding regions. In West and Central Africa, many migrants who cross borders for seasonal work were left stranded due to border closures during the pandemic. Humanitarian disasters fueled by violence, competition over natural resources, underdevelopment, and poverty in the Central Sahel region have resulted in the internal displacement of 1.9 million persons, and 106,701 confirmed deaths in Africa in 2020.

Asia

Asian countries initiated early mobility restrictions in 2020 to prevent the spread of the COVID-19 virus. These were quarantine measures, banning of arrivals, and border closures. Health measures increased over time. In addition to quarantine measures and health screening and monitoring, testing/medical certificate requirements were put into place.

Displacement is characteristic of this global region. In 2020, the top origin countries of refugees were the Syrian Arab Republic and Afghanistan. Turkey hosted more than 3.6 million refugees, with Pakistan and the Islamic Republic of Iran hosting approximately 2.6 million refugees from Afghanistan. Myanmar, another origin country of refugees, saw the largest number of persons flee, mainly the Rohingya, who were victims of violence and persecution. Many of the Rohingya are hosted in Bangladesh.

Internal displacements due to natural disasters add to humanitarian crises in regions where political conflict occurs. Flooding caused by monsoons, landslides, and intense cyclones account for the following approximate displacement of persons in 2020: Bangladesh (4 million), China (5 million), India (4 million), Philippines (4 million), and Vietnam (1 million).

East Asia

Migrants from this subregion experienced xenophobia and discrimination. This was also true for descendants of this subregion living in other parts of the world. Persons thought to be of Chinese descent were physically assaulted. Discriminatory practices in the subregion were quarantine requirements, mask rationing, and inaccessibility to social benefits and government subsidies. Many migrants were unable to return to their home countries due to travel restrictions.

Southeast Asia

Countries in this subregion instituted travel restrictions that included limiting public transportation and domestic flights, quarantine, testing, and border closures. The Philippines reported 1.4 million COVID cases in 2020. Crowded quarantine conditions increased the risk of persons contracting COVID-19. Jobless migrant workers hurried to return to their origin countries of Cambodia, Myanmar, and the Lao People's Democratic Republic while still able to do so. Nurses from the Philippines with contracts in other countries were immobilized due to travel restrictions.

Middle East

Migrants in the Middle East were significantly challenged by the pandemic. Travel and movement restrictions and border closures exacerbated existing health conditions and increased the risk of contracting COVID-19. Migrants were not routinely included in vaccination campaigns in countries where they were stranded. Risk factors included crowded living conditions, the nature of their work, and inadequate access to health care. With countries locked down and forced closure of company operations, many migrants lost jobs or had delayed wages. Ultimately, this affected their ability to meet basic needs, pay debts, and support those such as family or extended family who relied on them.

Europe

Europe saw an increase in international migrants numbering from 75 million in 2015 to 87 million in 2020. Large migrant populations reside in the Russian Federation (11 million), Ukraine (6 million), Poland (4.8 million), and Romania (84,330). Germany reportedly had 16 million migrants in 2020 from Poland, Turkey, the Russian Federation, Kazakhstan, and the Syrian Arab Republic. The following other countries in the European region report high numbers of migrants: United Kingdom (9.4 million), France (8.5 million), Spain (6.8 million), and Italy (6.4 million). As with other global regions, travel restrictions, including internal movement; quarantine; and health measures were in place during the pandemic.

Latin America and the Caribbean

In 2020, 25 million people from Latin America and the Caribbean have migrated to North America. This represents an increase from approximately 10 million persons in 1990. The political situation in Venezuela has led to approximately 5.6 million Venezuelans leaving in 2021, and about 4.6 million have moved to other Latin American countries (Columbia, Peru, Chile, Ecuador, and Brazil) and the Caribbean.

In spite of movement to North America, the top countries of emigres are Mexico (1,169,883; Integral Human Development, n.d.), Venezuela (5 million), and Columbia (3 million). Internal and international travel restrictions and quarantines were in place in 2020. As new waves of infection occurred in late 2020 and early 2021, restrictions were maintained.

Northern America

Canada and the United States are the main migration countries in Northern America. Nearly 59 million migrants resided in Northern America in 2020, mainly in the United States. Most migrants to Northern America were from Latin America and the Caribbean (26 million), Asia (18 million), and Europe (7 million). Factors influencing migration to Northern America are economic growth and political stability.

During the pandemic, internal and international controls were quickly put in place, with international travel restrictions instituted very early. Restrictions included screening measures and quarantine measures, border closures, and ban on arrivals from some regions. However, unlike other global regions, Northern American countries did not impose restrictions on general internal movement. Initially, during the early pandemic stages, there were more travel restrictions than health measures. Eventually, health measures exceeded travel measures.

Oceania

Nearly 8.3 million international migrants lived in Oceania in 2020. The majority of migrants lived in Australia and New Zealand. Internal and international movement restrictions were quickly put in place, with border closures, screening and ban on arrivals, and quarantine measures. Health-related measures were gradually put in place in the early months of the pandemic. Internal and global travel restrictions were greater than health-related measures by 2021.

To Stay or Leave: Factors Influencing Migration

Migration is a complex phenomenon. Resultant impacts of migration may be short-term or prolonged indefinitely. Consequently, migration may have significant, intergenerational consequences. Ready access to resources to maintain basic needs, health, and well-being are compromised. Education, gainful employment and living wages, safe housing and environments, and future planning are seemingly out of reach or suspended in uncertainty. Human connectedness to family, friends, support networks, and community are severely disrupted or lost altogether.

The contexts of migration are equally complex and vary widely. People migrate to reunify and maintain connectedness with family, relatives, and significant others.

The economic opportunity for gainful employment and better wages is another factor in migration. Many persons who have migrated for economic reasons are often the sole providers of financial support for family members remaining in their countries of origin. A stable environment or a better environment that supports healthy living and quality of life and provides educational opportunities is another reason for migration. Environmental factors, political conflict, safety, and security are other drivers of migration.

Economic Factors and Work Programs

People migrate for economic reasons. Countries offer work programs, as noted previously, that attract and retain a multinational workforce. Better wages, steady employment, and job advancement may draw people across borders. While the economic opportunities offer appeal and financial stability, including the increased ability to send remittances to family, this may come at the expense of being away from family and home many months at a time. Unless work programs abroad also integrate extended family leave time, meaningful cultural-social activities, and effective work relationships, there is the potential for diminishing mental health and well-being, social isolation, and depression in persons who migrate across borders for employment.

Human Development

Migration also occurs for the purposes of human development. Matching knowledge and skill sets to meet labor demands or to fulfill a lack or deficit of human resources in other regions is a reason for migration. Education, training, and exchange programs to acquire or provide experience, expertise, and skills may be long-term or short-term, temporary, or permanent.

Sociocultural

Family unification or reunification is another impetus for migration. Individuals or groups may choose to migrate and resettle in a particular region with others of like ethnicity and cultural background. A shared understanding of common beliefs, values, and traditions help create community.

Environmental

Another driver of migration is risks or threats to habitability resulting from climate change and environmental and natural disasters. Multiple factors contribute to domestic movement or cross-border movement. Extreme environmental events affect health, income, food security, water supply, and human security. Drought-stricken regions experience poor agricultural yields, decreased income, and increased deprivation. Dwindling resources and competition for resources may create tensions and conflict in affected regions. Poorer households in highly exposed locations are at risk. These households may not have the means to move and become further impoverished and trapped in place. Internal migration across developing countries projected to 2050 is expected to range from 44 million to 216 million people under different climate, demographic, and developmental scenarios (World Bank, 2023, p. 78).

Conflict

Political and armed conflict is one example of a safety and security issue that has led to migration. Under such circumstances, escaping these events is often unplanned and without clear, organized, or safe pathways to a destination point. Important identity documents may be left behind, which can be a source of burden and further vulnerability in meeting basic needs, seeking aid, or gaining access to health care. Persons fleeing armed conflict and violence may leave with little resources or expend all financial resources for safe transport at the risk of vulnerability to ill-intended others who illicitly victimize persons in an emergent situation.

Migration from an origin point such as one's home, place of residence, or community to a destination safety point is varied. The decision to leave may be unquestionable and clear in the presence of an immediate threat to life and safety. For others, such as older adults, who have firm roots in a place or who are without family, relatives, or close friends they may rely on for assistance, the decision to relocate and leave may be fraught with indecision, anxiety, and fear for a future of uncertainty and instability. Internal displacement occurs by moving from one location to another within country borders for safety and security reasons. External displacement occurs when crossing an international border, also for safety and security reasons. Fear of persecution is a significant factor that leads people to seek international protection, refuge, or asylum in another country. Persons migrating for these reasons are caught in peril as host governments debate entry, resources, and relocation or lack clear infrastructure, processes, and support.

Refugees, Asylum Seekers, Displaced Persons

The United Nations Office of the High Commissioner for Refugees (UNHCR) "leads international action in protecting people forced to flee conflict and persecution and those denied a nationality" (UNHCR, n.d.). According to a UNHCR report on global trends, 108.4 million persons were forcibly displaced worldwide at the end of 2022 (UNHCR, 2023; Figure 6.4). Persecution, conflict, violence, human rights violations,

Children account for 30 percent of the world's population, but 40 percent of forcibly displaced people.*

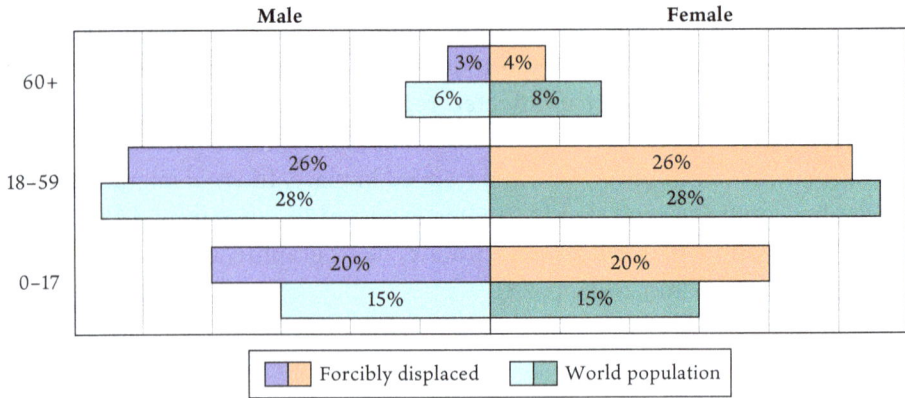

FIGURE 6.4   Demographics of People Who Have Been Forcibly Displaced

or serious disturbances of public order led to displacement. Among those displaced were 35.3 million refugees, 62.5 million internally displaced persons, 5.4 million asylum seekers, and 5.2 million other people in need of international protection. The latter is defined as persons who are outside their country or territory of origin who have been forcibly displaced across international borders and who have not been reported categorically as asylum seekers, refugees, and in refugee-like situations but likely need international protection. This includes protection against forced return and access to basic services on a temporary or long-term basis (UNHCR, 2023).

The UNHCR reports that in 2022, low- and middle-income countries hosted 76% of refugees and people in need of protection, with the least developed countries providing asylum to 20% of the total forcibly displaced persons. In addition, 70% of refugees and others needing international protection were hosted in countries neighboring origin countries. In 2022, 52% of refugees and others needing international protection came from three countries, the Syrian Arab Republic (6.5 million), Ukraine (5.7 million), and Afghanistan (5.7 million). The UNHCR resettled a total of 114,300 refugees. Internally displaced persons and refugees who returned to their areas or countries of origin numbered 6 million. Data also shows that 7% of forcibly displaced persons are older adults aged 60 years or older (Figure 6.4).

Refugee crises continue to grow. According to the World Development Report (World Bank, 2023), the number of refugees has doubled in the last decade. In mid-2022, the UNHCR reported 37.8 million refugees worldwide with 26.7 million refugees and persons in refugee-like situations, 5.8 million Palestinians, and 5.3 million in need of international protection. In addition, 4.9 million asylum seekers await a decision. As of February 2023, 8 million refugees fled to neighboring countries, and 5.4 million are internally displaced (World Bank, 2023).

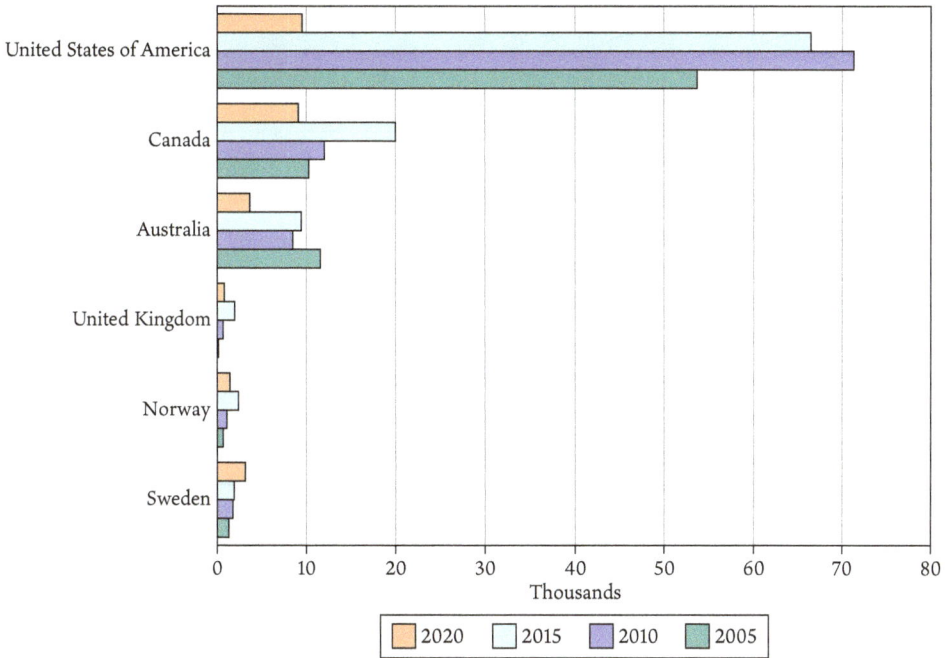

FIGURE 6.5 Number of Refugees Resettled by Major Resettlement Country in 2005–2020

There is little disaggregated data about older adult refugees and their plight. Intertwining factors, such as health status; psychosocial, cultural, or socioeconomic circumstances; and issues of resettlement affect the decision to stay or flee. Older adults with functional limitations, disability, or chronic illness may not have the strength or stamina to withstand the physical activities of relocation. Access to health care professionals, ongoing care, medications, or treatment may be inadequate or absent for an undetermined amount of time. Psychosocial factors involve family ties, social support, and community networks. Family separation and loss of social support networks for tangible material aid, emotional support, and psychosocial support generate significant trauma and stress. Language and communication are important aspects of culture. Being without the ability to communicate and to be understood in one's native or preferred language is an additional stressor and hardship further compounding relocation, whether under duress or forced relocation. Women and girls of all ages have special health and protection needs, and these are often unmet and unheeded. They are frequently subject to exploitation. Women-headed households are particularly challenged, with limited access to the labor market, education, and adequate health services (World Bank, 2023, p. 209; Figure 6.3). Concerns about income and gainful employment to support oneself or one's family is a socioeconomic issue. The ability to use one's skill sets to maintain self-sufficiency once resettled is an uncertainty. The loss of assets, coupled with traumatic ordeals and limited access to opportunities, leads to poverty.

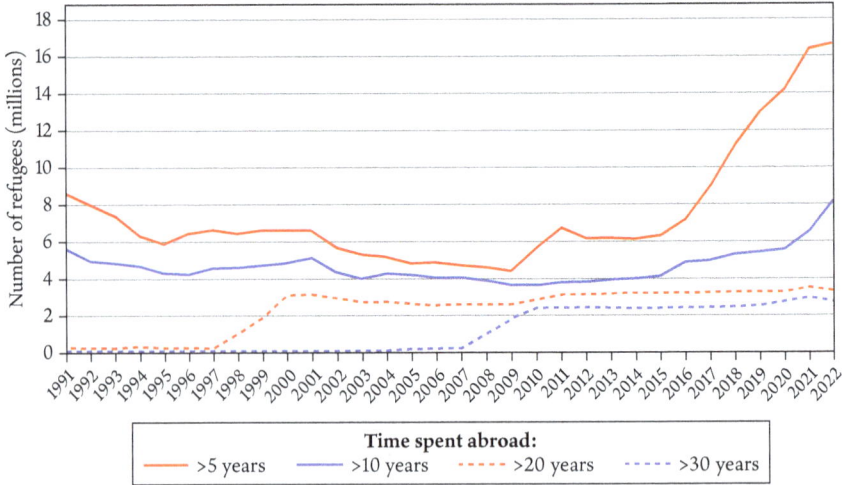

Note: Data for 2022 are as of mid-2022, when the latest figures were available.

FIGURE 6.5   Refugees in Protracted Situations

Relocation and resettlement of refugees may be a short-term or protracted indefinite process. This in itself creates undue stress, and the mental health challenges of refugees are well documented in the literature. Statistics from the UNHCR database indicate that refugees in protracted situations have more than doubled over the last decade (World Bank, 2023, p. 209; Figure 6.5).

International Agreements and Global Compact: Solutions

There have been several major agreements among nation-states to achieve critical objectives to safeguard migrant lives during movement, transition, and resettlement, as well as their health and well-being. These international agreements are the Strategic Plan of the International Organization for Migration (IOM, 2024), the New York Declaration for Refugees and Migrants (United Nations, 2016), the Global Compact for Safe, Orderly, and Regular Migration (United Nations, 2019), the World Health Organization Draft Global Action Plan 2019–2023 (WHO, 2019a), and Expectations, Gaps, Perspectives (WHO, 2019b).

The Strategic Plan of the IOM (2024) defines infrastructure among nation-states for achievement of three objectives:

- Saving lives and protecting people on the move
- Driving solutions to displacement
- Facilitating pathways for regular migration

The New York Declaration (United Nations, 2016) served as a precursory document to the Global Compact (United Nations, 2019). The New York Declaration is a statement of political will and commitments to address the question of large movements of refugees and migrants. International cooperation, accurate information, protection of human rights and fundamental freedoms, health care needs, integration and inclusion, and education are among the declared commitments. The Global Compact further delineates agreements of nation-states to the achievement of 23 objectives (Table 6.4) and their implementation, follow-up, and review. Several guiding principles are the foundation of the Global Compact:

- People-centered
- International cooperation
- National sovereignty
- Rule of law and due process
- Sustainable development
- Human rights
- Gender-responsive
- Child-sensitive
- Whole-of-government approach
- Whole-of-society approach

TABLE 6.4 Objectives for Safe, Orderly, and Regular Migration

1. Collect and utilize accurate and disaggregated data as a basis for evidence-based policies
2. Minimize the adverse drivers and structural factors that compel people to leave their country of origin
3. Provide accurate and timely information at all stages of migration
4. Ensure that all migrants have proof of legal identity and adequate documentation
5. Enhance availability and flexibility of pathways for regular migration
6. Facilitate fair and ethical recruitment and safeguard conditions that ensure decent work
7. Address and reduce vulnerabilities in migration
8. Save lives and establish coordinated international efforts on missing migrants
9. Strengthen the transnational response
10. Prevent, combat and eradicate trafficking in persons in the context of international migration

11. Manage borders in an integrated, secure and coordinated manner

12. Strengthen certainty and predictability in migration procedures for appropriate screening, assessment and referral

13. Use migration detention only as a measure of last resort and work towards alternatives

14. Enhance consular protection, assistance and cooperation throughout the migration cycle

15. Provide access to basic services for migrants

16. Empower migrants and societies to realize full inclusion and social cohesion

17. Eliminate all forms of discrimination and promote evidence-based public discourse to shape perceptions of migration

18. Invest in skills development and facilitate mutual recognition of skills, qualifications and competencies

19. Create conditions for migrants and diasporas to fully contribute to sustainable development in all countries

20. Promote faster, safer and cheaper transfer of remittances and foster financial inclusion of migrants

21. Cooperate in facilitating safe and dignified return and readmission, as well as sustainable reintegration

22. Establish mechanisms for the portability of social security entitlements and earned benefits

23. Strengthen international cooperation and global partnerships for safe, orderly and regular migration

Source: United Nations General Assembly Global Compact for Safe, Orderly and Regular Migration (United Nations, 2019). https://www.un.org/en/development/desa/population/migration/generalassembly/docs/globalcompact/A_RES_73_195.pdf

Nation-states of the United Nations through the Global Compact for Safe, Orderly and Regular Migration (United Nations, 2019) have agreed to the following actions:

Incorporate the health needs of migrants into national and local health-care policies and plans, such as by strengthening capacities for service provision, facilitating affordable and non-discriminatory access, reducing communication barriers, and training health-care providers on culturally sensitive service delivery, in order to promote the physical and mental health of migrants and communities overall, including by taking into consideration relevant recommendations from the World Health Organization Framework of Guiding Principles to Promote the Health of Refugees and Migrants.

Nonetheless, although a global compact exists, access to health care and social protection services remains very limited and requires out-of-pocket expenditures, which quickly deplete personal resources and tip individuals and families into poverty. International compacts and laws do not uphold the rights of older persons. Inconvenient locations and long distances to reach health care services, language barriers, and discrimination continue to be problematic. Persons seeking refuge, protection services, and those who are displaced are frequently mass-housed indefinitely in "temporary" shelters that lack basic conditions for handwashing, personal hygiene and privacy, and sanitation services for waste elimination and management. Contamination and transmission of infectious diseases readily occur in densely populated shelters with poor ventilation. Migrants may be forced to live and travel through unsheltered conditions with little protection against the elements.

Food insecurity and access to nutritious foods sufficient to meet the needs of older adults is an ongoing concern. Related issues are sanitary spaces and essential equipment for food preparation and food storage. Women often bear the burden of collecting water and gathering firewood for cooking and heating. These tasks require walking at length to distant and remote areas, and unfortunately, women are also targeted and subject to physical violence.

Men in migration are subject to physical violence, torture, and imprisonment. Men, women, persons with diverse gender identities (WHO, 2022), and persons with disabilities in migration have difficulty accessing health care and face discrimination (Inter-Agency Standing Committee [IASC], 2019).

Migration data for older adults has not been accurately tracked or addressed in policy decisions, programs, and protection services. The World Health Organization (2022) reports that in fragile countries facing the likelihood of increasing conflict and disasters, the proportion of people aged 50 years or older is projected to increase from 12.3% (219.9 million) in 2020 to 19.2% (586.3 million) in 2050. Interviews in 2019 conducted across 11 countries during humanitarian crises (African region, Eastern Mediterranean, Americas) found that 77% of the older people interviewed lacked income, 64% lacked food, and 25% had no access to clean water. Women were disproportionately affected. Among the older adult women interviewees, 58% were living alone, 56% were caring for others, 56% had no access to health care, 58% had no access to food, and 58% had no income (McGivern et al., 2020).

Older adults encounter exclusion and discrimination. Among the interviewees in the 2019 study, 77% indicated they had not been asked by any other humanitarian agency about the services being provided to them. Of those interviewed, 63% were caring for at least one child, and 44% were caring for another older person. The absence of basic services (housing, food, nutrition, and health care) and the absence of traditional and family support systems exacerbate any existing health issues and increase their vulnerability for health deterioration.

Health literacy is a critical determinant of health. Low levels of health literacy combined with language barriers affect seeking of, and access to, health care services and treatment adherence. Culturally sensitive, age-appropriate interpretation services and translation of health promotion materials can improve health literacy. Health literacy is vital for screening, illness prevention, risk and chronic illness management, and prevention of occupational and home hazards (WHO, 2022).

Through an Ethical Lens: Perspectives on the Health Care of Older Adult Migrants

The interplay of ethical practice, migration of older adults, and health care services is multifaceted and requires collaboration at the intersections of culture, accountability of government to its citizenry, inclusive policies, and financial sustainability. The intent of this section is to raise awareness of complex issues and thereby generate solutions within one's circle of immediate influence.

As discussed previously, ageism and age discrimination are a pervasive global issue. Older adults' worth to society is devalued. Older adults may be viewed as economically burdensome to families. Older adults contend with chronic illness, loss of income, and diminished social support networks and may have only remaining family to turn to for assistance. The voices of older adults are often excluded from policy-making decisions and legislation. Therefore, they are an excluded and marginalized group who are left without social and health protections. Resource allocation for older adults in migration or resettlement are the least priority in local governments, in spite of international compacts. The absence of priority services to migrant populations allows for exploitation and illicit activities at many levels, which include smugglers who deprive persons of their personal assets and human labor and sex traffickers. Wage theft among laborers in various industries is a growing concern.

Costs of treatment and medications, along with unfathomable, complicated health insurance requirements, are a deterrent to many who are unable to access care. The COVID-19 pandemic proved that health care infrastructure and the preparedness of health care professional staff were woefully inadequate on a global scale.

- Is health care truly a basic human right, as are adequate nutrition, safe drinking water, adequate shelter, and clean air?

- How can vaccines, medications, and evidence-based treatments be delivered to all persons in a timely manner regardless of personal income or country income level and geographic region?

- What are strategies through which older adult voices and health concerns can be authentically and directly heard so that health care systems are responsive to their needs in their respective communities?

- How are health care systems responding to the health care needs of older adults in the context of their respective communities?

- How is this response sustained, evaluated, and changed as needed over time?

- How do health care systems ensure an integrated response (vs. a fragmented one) to older adult care as their needs change over time?

- To what extent do older adult voices inform and shape decisions and policies?

- To what extent are health care policies inclusive or exclusive of issues affecting older adults?

The immediate and long-term health consequences of delayed or absent care for older adult migrant populations comes at a human cost—death resulting from preventable illness and disease, a downward spiraling of health, or lost capacity and productivity to society, which could have contributed to the betterment of families and communities, as well as further loss of immediate support networks. Human suffering encompasses not only the physical but also the mental, emotional, and spiritual aspects of well-being.

Interpersonal and Transcultural Caregiving Skills

Building trust and respecting the other's perspective while attempting to acquire entre to persons or groups who are migrating, relocating, or resettling is essential to caregiving and provision of services. Asking questions about another's concerns, without preformulating a response, facilitates uninhibited expression of needs and priorities, both immediate and long-term.

Inquiry into normal patterns of daily living, traditional health practices, and Indigenous beliefs about health, wellness, and illness build trust while acquiring valuable assessments (Leininger, 2006; Clark et al., 2009; Kleinman et al., 1978). At the point of care, inquiry about understanding of illness, the decision-making process, and acceptable interventions may pave the way for negotiation or repatterning health behaviors (for example, is hypertension or high blood pressure an understood concept, who makes health care decisions, who is consulted within the family, which treatments or interventions are unacceptable based on values or religious beliefs).

Engaging the older adult in all phases of their care may take time and commitment—explaining, interpreting, assessing, treating, evaluating, renegotiating, and repatterning or establishing new health behaviors. This can be a daunting task for older adults and health care professionals, but nonetheless essential and worthwhile. As much as possible, detailed medical record documentation should be provided to the older adult in migration. Having the documentation will allow for some continuity of care in movement from one place to another.

Persons in resettlement need vital, direct, and immediate connections to resources to meet basic needs. These include adequate housing, ready access to health care, nutrition, employment or a source of income, education, transportation, and social support networks, as they create a sense of stability and reestablish a sense of community and belonging.

A comprehensive assessment tool, developed by the author, *Care Seeking in Resettlement: A Nursing Screening and Health Assessment Tool* (Catolico, 2013), identifies priorities among persons in resettlement. The tool was developed from a qualitative research study and a review of the literature. The tool's survey to be asked of persons in resettlement consists of eight domains, each with operational definitions:

Domain 1: Migration-displacement-transition experience

Domain 2: Resettlement (subdomains include housing, health, relationships, transportation, and work)

Domain 3: Socioeconomic status

Domain 4: Social supports

Domain 5: Neighborhood characteristics

Domain 6: Health knowledge and practices

Domain 7: Access to care

Domain 8: Perceived discrimination

To date, the tool has been piloted with a panel of nurse experts to determine its content validity. The content validity index (CVI) measures scale relevance and ranges from 0.00 (item irrelevant) to 1.00 (item highly relevant). The CVI for scale relevance of the Care Seeking in Resettlement tool is 0.866 overall. Although further studies using this tool with persons in resettlement are needed, the tool may serve as a launching point to connect people with vital services (Appendix A).

Chapter Summary

This chapter has provided an overview of migration trends and factors influencing migration. Little data exist on older adults in migration, although aging societies exist in many world regions. Older adults are the most vulnerable and at the greatest risk for health consequences related to migration and other socioeconomic-environmental factors.

Appendix A: Care-Seeking in Resettlement: A Nursing Screening and Health Assessment Tool

Definition of terms:

Person in resettlement: An individual who has experienced migration, displacement, or transition, irrespective of time in any location, geographical distances, and country borders, and who has been in the U.S. for up to 7 years.

Health care encounter: a nursing interaction, (initial, episodic, or continuous), <u>with</u> individuals for the purposes of assessment, intervention, treatment, advisement and education, or referral to another healthcare professional, service, or organization for follow-up care, continuity in care, or specialty consultation. The modes of interaction include an actual face-to-face encounter (in person), virtual (video teleconferencing, web-based), electronic (email, chat), or phone.

Cultural sensitivity: the fostering of therapeutic interaction, communication, attentiveness, respect for differences (beliefs, values, behaviors).

Cultural safety: nonjudgmental interactions that freely permit expression of individual and/or group identity.

In consideration of the totality and intensity of the migration experiences of persons in resettlement, the researcher developed questions instead of statements. Questions may better facilitate cultural sensitivity and safety through nurse-to-individual interaction, in place of impersonal statements on a form to mark. Questions allow for expression of individual perspective and meaning in one's own words.

Registered Nurse (RN) participants were asked to rate each of the questions, *to be asked of persons in resettlement* during a healthcare encounter, based on their *relevance* and *clarity*. Please use the definition terminologies that are provided.

Relevance is the applicability or pertinence to the measured domain. The response options denote the following, 4= the item is highly relevant to the measured domain, 3= the item is quite relevant to the measured domain, 2= the item is somewhat relevant to the measured domain, 1= the item is not relevant to the measured domain.

Clarity is the transparency or clearness of items under each domain. The response options denote the following, 4= the item is clear, 3= the item needs minor revisions, 2= the item needs major revisions to be clear, 1= the item is not clear.

There are 8 domains, with questions pertaining to each domain. Participants may enter open ended comments, suggestions, or revisions.

CARE-SEEKING IN RESETTLEMENT: A NURSING SCREENING AND HEALTH ASSESSMENT TOOL

Domain One: Migration-Displacement-Transition Experience

Definition:

The act of having to uproot, migrate, move, from a place of stability, or one's permanent place of residence to another, whether temporary, or longer-term, regardless of length of time spent in any one location, and regardless of geographical distances and country borders between moves. The individual determines what is considered as a place of stability, or their permanent place of residence. The migration experience encompasses all of what the person experienced. Therefore, questions statements are included about circumstance, safety, health and illness, and treatment.

Question	Relevance to the domain 4=highly relevant 3=quite relevant 2=somewhat relevant 1=not relevant				Clarity of the question 4=clear 3=needs minor revisions 2=needs major revision 1=not clear			
	4	3	2	1	4	3	2	1
1. What situation led to your decision to leave your permanent place of residence?	○	○	○	○	○	○	○	○
2. What kind of work did you do prior to leaving your permanent place of residence?	○	○	○	○	○	○	○	○
3. Were you separated from others who were with you as you moved from one place to another?	○	○	○	○	○	○	○	○
4. Have you lived in more than one temporary or transitional space?	○	○	○	○	○	○	○	○

Question	4	3	2	1	4	3	2	1
5. How much time was spent living in temporary or transitional spaces each time you moved from one place to another? (shelter, refugee camp, detention center)?	○	○	○	○	○	○	○	○
6. What were your major concerns as you moved from one place to another?	○	○	○	○	○	○	○	○
7. Were you concerned for your safety as you moved from one place to another?	○	○	○	○	○	○	○	○
8. What did you do to stay safe as you moved from one place to another?	○	○	○	○	○	○	○	○
9. What major health problems or illnesses did you experience while in these transitional spaces?	○	○	○		○	○	○	○

Domain One: Migration-Displacement-Transition Experience

Definition:
The act of having to uproot, migrate, move, from a place of stability, or one's permanent place of residence to another, whether temporary, or longer-term, regardless of length of time spent in any one location, and regardless of geographical distances and country borders between moves. The individual determines what is considered as a place of stability, or their permanent place of residence. The migration experience encompasses all of what the person experienced. Therefore, questions statements are included about circumstance, safety, health and illness, and treatment.

Question	Relevance to the domain 4=highly relevant 3=quite relevant 2=somewhat relevant 1=not relevant				Clarity of the question 4=clear 3=needs minor revisions 2=needs major revision 1=not clear			
	4	3	2	1	4	3	2	1
10. What treatments were you given for your health problems or illnesses while in transition?	○	○	○	○	○	○	○	○
11. Did your health problems or illnesses improve after treatment?	○	○	○	○	○	○	○	○
12. Were you able to get help for other major concerns you had while in transition?	○	○	○	○	○	○	○	○

Comments about the domain migration-displacement-transition:

Comments about the question items:

Domain Two: Resettlement

Definition: *Resettlement is the process of making necessary life adjustments to regain or maintain stability, post-migration, as described by the individual. Necessary life adjustments in resettlement consists of other subdomains in resettlement which are housing, health, relationships, transportation, and work.*

Question	Relevance to the domain				Clarity of the question			
	4=highly relevant 3=quite relevant 2=somewhat relevant 1=not relevant				4=clear 3=needs minor revisions 2=needs major revision 1=not clear			
	4	3	2	1	4	3	2	1
	○	○	○	○	○	○	○	○

Subdomain: Housing in Resettlement
Definition: *for this study, housing is the individual's current place of residence*

13. How would you describe the quality of your current living situation with respect to the following areas below:

	4	3	2	1	4	3	2	1
a. Sleeping space?	○	○	○	○	○	○	○	○
b. Food storage and preparation areas?	○	○	○	○	○	○	○	○
c. Bathroom area?	○	○	○	○	○	○	○	○
d. Plumbing?	○	○	○	○	○	○	○	○

Question	Relevance				Clarity			
	4	3	2	1	4	3	2	1
e. Safe drinking water?	○	○	○	○	○	○	○	○
f. Electricity?	○	○	○	○	○	○	○	○
g. Presence of other hazardous physical conditions?	○	○	○	○	○	○	○	○
14. Do you feel safe in your house?	○	○	○	○	○	○	○	○

Comments about the subdomain housing:

Domain Two: Resettlement

Definition: *Resettlement is the process of making necessary life adjustments to regain or maintain stability, post-migration, as described by the individual. Necessary life adjustments in resettlement consists of other subdomains in resettlement which are housing, health, relationships, transportation, and work.*

Relevance to the domain
4=highly relevant
3=quite relevant
2=somewhat relevant
1=not relevant

Clarity of the question
4=clear
3=needs minor revisions
2=needs major revision
1=not clear

Comments about the question items:

Domain Two: Resettlement

Definition: *Resettlement is the process of making necessary life adjustments to regain or maintain stability, post-migration, as described by the individual. Necessary life adjustments in resettlement consists of other subdomains in resettlement which are housing, health, relationships, transportation, and work.*

Question:

	Relevance to the domain 4=highly relevant 3=quite relevant 2=somewhat relevant 1=not relevant				Clarity of the question 4=clear 3=needs minor revisions 2=needs major revision 1=not clear			
	4	3	2	1	4	3	2	1
	○	○	○	○	○	○	○	○

Subdomain: Health

Definition: for this study, health in resettlement is the individual's expression of their geneal state of personal well-being or infirmity, whether physical, mental, or psychosocial. Health knowledge and practices, and access to care are assessments that (are separately addressed in other domains, 6 and 7)

	4	3	2	1	4	3	2	1
15. How would you describe your overall health now?	4 ○	3 ○	2 ○	1 ○	4 ○	3 ○	2 ○	1 ○
16. Does your health seem better than before?	4 ○	3 ○	2 ○	1 ○	4 ○	3 ○	2 ○	1 ○
17. Does your health seem worse than before?	4 ○	3 ○	2 ○	1 ○	4 ○	3 ○	2 ○	1 ○
18. What are the reasons that account for your overall health now?	4 ○	3 ○	2 ○	1 ○	4 ○	3 ○	2 ○	1 ○
19. Are you experiencing health problems that you have not experienced before?	4 ○	3 ○	2 ○	1 ○	4 ○	3 ○	2 ○	1 ○
20. What are your major health concerns at this time?	4 ○	3 ○	2 ○	1 ○	4 ○	3 ○	2 ○	1 ○

Comments about the subdomain health:

Comments about the question items:

Domain Two: Resettlement

Definition: *Resettlement is the process of making necessary life adjustments to regain or maintain stability, post-migration, as described by the individual. Necessary life adjustments in resettlement consists of other subdomains in resettlement which are housing, health, relationships, transportation, and work.*

Question	Relevance to the domain 4=highly relevant 3=quite relevant 2=somewhat relevant 1=not relevant				Clarity of the question 4=clear 3=needs minor revisions 2=needs major revision 1=not clear			
	4	3	2	1	4	3	2	1
	○	○	○	○	○	○	○	○

Subdomain: Relationships in Resettlement

Definition: *for this study, relationships are family relationships as identified by the individual; the nature of the migration experience, whether brief or prolonged, redefine family constitution as relationships develop, emerge, evolve, or change. The individual determines who constitutes family relationships (for ex: nuclear or immediate family, blended family, relatives, extended family, domestic partnerships).*

Question	4	3	2	1	4	3	2	1
21. Who are the people in your family?	○	○	○	○	○	○	○	○
22. How often do you see one another?	○	○	○	○	○	○	○	○
23. How do you spend your time together?	○	○	○	○	○	○	○	○

24. What are special celebrations in your family?

4 ○ 3 ○ 2 ○ 1 ○   4 ○ 3 ○ 2 ○ 1 ○

25. What opportunities have happened within your family?

4 ○ 3 ○ 2 ○ 1 ○   4 ○ 3 ○ 2 ○ 1 ○

26. What setbacks have happened within your family?

4 ○ 3 ○ 2 ○ 1 ○   4 ○ 3 ○ 2 ○ 1 ○

27. To what extent do family members rely upon one another to help care for other members? (for example: caring for young children while away at work, caring for an ill family member, caring for a frail elderly member)

4 ○ 3 ○ 2 ○ 1 ○   4 ○ 3 ○ 2 ○ 1 ○

28. How would you describe your relationship with your family?

4 ○ 3 ○ 2 ○ 1 ○   4 ○ 3 ○ 2 ○ 1 ○

Comments about the subdomain relationships:

Comments about the question items:

Domain Two: Resettlement

Definition: *Resettlement is the process of making necessary life adjustments to regain or maintain stability post-migration, as described by the individual. Necessary life adjustments in resettlement consists of other subdomains in resettlement which are housing, health, relationships, transportation, and work.*

Question	Relevance to the domain 4=highly relevant 3=quite relevant 2=somewhat relevant 1=not relevant				Clarity of the question 4=clear 3=needs minor revisions 2=needs major revision 1=not clear			
	4	3	2	1	4	3	2	1
	○	○	○	○	○	○	○	○

Subdomain: Transportation in Resettlement

Definition: *transportation refers to the ability to travel from one place to another for the purposes of daily living (work, school, grocery shopping, healthcare, recreation, socialization)*

Question	4	3	2	1	4	3	2	1
29. How does ready access to personal transportation affect your ability to get around in your community?	○	○	○	○	○	○	○	○
30. What do you do for transportation in the community where you live now?	○	○	○	○	○	○	○	○
31. How do you get to work?	○	○	○	○	○	○	○	○
32. How do your children get to school?	○	○	○	○	○	○	○	○
33. How do you get to the grocery store?	○	○	○	○	○	○	○	○

Domain Two: Resettlement

Definition: *Resettlement is the process of making necessary life adjustments to regain or maintain stability, post-migration, as described by the individual. Necessary life adjustments in resettlement consists of other subdomains in resettlement which are <u>housing, health, relationships, transportation, and work</u>.*

Question	Relevance to the domain 4=highly relevant 3=quite relevant 2=somewhat relevant 1=not relevant				Clarity of the question 4=clear 3=needs minor revisions 2=needs major revision 1=not clear			
	4	3	2	1	4	3	2	1
	○	○	○	○	○	○	○	○

Subdomain: Transportation in Resettlement

Definition: *transportation refers to the ability to travel from one place to another for the purposes of daily living (work, school, grocery shopping, healthcare, recreation, socialization)*

Question	4	3	2	1	4	3	2	1
34. How do you get to any appointments you may have?	○	○	○	○	○	○	○	○
35. How often do you rely upon family, relatives, or friends to provide needed transportation?	○	○	○	○	○	○	○	○
36. How often do you rely upon public transportation?	○	○	○	○	○	○	○	○
37. To what extent does access to personal transportation affect recreational activity?	○	○	○	○	○	○	○	○
38. To what extent does access to personal transportation affect socialization with family, relatives, and friends?	○	○	○	○	○	○	○	○

Comments about the subdomain transportation:

Comments about question items:

Domain Two: Resettlement

Definition: Resettlement is the process of making necessary life adjustments to regain or maintain stability, post-migration, as described by the individual. Necessary life adjustments in resettlement consists of other subdomains in resettlement which are housing, health, relationships, transportation, and work.

Relevance to the domain
4=highly relevant
3=quite relevant
2=somewhat relevant
1=not relevant

Clarity of the question
4=clear
3=needs minor revisions
2=needs major revision
1=not clear

Subdomain: Work in Resettlement
Definition: work is the means, process, use of knowl families edge, skills, abilities, by which persons earn money to support themselves, families

Question	Relevance 4	3	2	1	Clarity 4	3	2	1
39. What is your current work situation?	○	○	○	○	○	○	○	○
40. How would you describe the working conditions where you currently work?	○	○	○	○	○	○	○	○
41. What new skills, knowledge, and abilities did you acquire for the work that you do now?	○	○	○	○	○	○	○	○
42. What skills, knowledge, and abilities did you already possess for the work that you do now?	○	○	○	○	○	○	○	○

Comments about the subdomain work:

Comments about the question items:

Domain Three: Socio-Economic Status

Definition: *Socioeconomic status is the individual's measure or judgment of their social and economic position, attributable to their work experience, income, occupation, and education.*

Question	Relevance to the domain 4=highly relevant 3=quite relevant 2=somewhat relevant 1=not relevant				Clarity of the question 4=clear 3=needs minor revisions 2=needs major revision 1=not clear			
	4	3	2	1	4	3	2	1
43. How would you describe your ability to provide for yourself and others who rely upon you?	○	○	○	○	○	○	○	○
44. What resources do you have to provide for yourself and others who rely upon you?	○	○	○	○	○	○	○	○
45. What worries you the most about not being able to provide adequately for yourself and others who rely upon you?	○	○	○	○	○	○	○	○
46. What do you consider as most *essential* resources that are needed at this time for yourself and others who rely upon you?	○	○	○	○	○	○	○	○
47. What would help you obtain upward economic mobility for yourself?	○	○	○	○	○	○	○	○
48. What would help you obtain upward economic mobility for yourself and others who rely upon you?	○	○	○	○	○	○	○	○

Comments about the domain socio-economic status:

Comments about the question items:

Domain Four: Social Supports

Definition: *Social support is the network of others, as identified by the individual, that provides tangible or intangible support, which is perceived to positively bolster the individual's capabilities and response to difficulties, as well as their strengths*

Question	Relevance to the domain 4=highly relevant 3=quite relevant 2=somewhat relevant 1=not relevant				Clarity of the question 4=clear 3=needs minor revisions 2=needs major revision 1=not clear			
	4	3	2	1	4	3	2	1
49. Generally, who are the people you rely upon for support and assistance in difficult times?	○	○	○	○	○	○	○	○
50. When you are faced with worries or troubles, who do you turn to first for help and assistance?	○	○	○	○	○	○	○	○
51. Who are other persons that will support you when you are troubled or worried?	○	○	○	○	○	○	○	○
52. When you are worried or troubled, how are people who support you helpful to you?	○	○	○	○	○	○	○	○
53. When you do not know what to do, who else do you turn to for help and assistance?	○	○	○	○	○	○	○	○
54. When you are working toward achieving something that is worthwhile to you, who are persons that support you in your efforts?	○	○	○	○	○	○	○	○

Comments about the domain social supports:

Comments about the question items:

Domain Five: Neighborhood Characteristics

Definition: *Neighborhood characteristics are those built community provisions and services in the environment in which the individual lives*

Question	Relevance to the domain 4=highly relevant 3=quite relevant 2=somewhat relevant 1=not relevant				Clarity of the question 4=clear 3=needs minor revisions 2=needs major revision 1=not clear			
	4	3	2	1	4	3	2	1
55. What is your neighborhood like?	○	○	○	○	○	○	○	○
56. How would you describe your neighborhood with respect to the following?								
a. A safe place for exercise and recreational activities?	○	○	○	○	○	○	○	○
b. How far is the closest school?	○	○	○	○	○	○	○	○
c. How far is the closet grocery store?	○	○	○	○	○	○	○	○
d. How far is the closest hospital?	○	○	○	○	○	○	○	○
e. How far is the nearest fire station?	○	○	○	○	○	○	○	○
f. Is there easy access to public transportation?	○	○	○	○	○	○	○	○
57. Are there disruptions in the provision of public utilities in the community where you live? (for example, electricity, natural gas, running water, safe drinking water)	○	○	○	○	○	○	○	○
58. Are there environmental hazards that pose a threat in the community where you live?	○	○	○	○	○	○	○	○

Domain Five: Neighborhood Characteristics

Definition: *Neighborhood characteristics are those built community provisions and services in the environment in which the individual lives*

Question	Relevance to the domain 4=highly relevant 3=quite relevant 2=somewhat relevant 1=not relevant				Clarity of the question 4=clear 3=needs minor revisions 2=needs major revision 1=not clear			
	4	3	2	1	4	3	2	1
59. What characteristics are the least likeable about the neighborhood in which you live?	○	○	○	○	○	○	○	○
60. What characteristics are most likeable about the neighborhood in which you live?	○	○	○	○	○	○	○	○

Comments about the domain neighborhood characteristics:

Comments about the question items:

Domain Six: Health Knowledge and Practices

Definition: *The individual's knowledge and understanding of health and illness, including utilization of indigenous health practices*

Question	Relevance to the domain 4=highly relevant 3=quite relevant 2=somewhat relevant 1=not relevant				Clarity of the question 4=clear 3=needs minor revisions 2=needs major revision 1=not clear			
	4	3	2	1	4	3	2	1
61. What do you do to stay well?	○	○	○	○	○	○	○	○
62. When you are ill, are there cultural expressions that describe what you are feeling or experiencing?	○	○	○	○	○	○	○	○
63. When you are ill, what traditional or cultural remedies do you use first to feel better before seeking help from a nurse or doctor?	○	○	○	○	○	○	○	○
64. When you are ill, are you able to describe your problem to the nurse or doctor?	○	○	○	○	○	○	○	○
65. When you are ill, do you feel your problems are understood by the nurse or doctor?	○	○	○	○	○	○	○	○
66. Are there feelings, thoughts, or experiences that trouble you for which there are no words to describe your problem to the nurse or doctor?	○	○	○	○	○	○	○	○

Comments about the domain health knowledge and practice:

Comments about the question items:

Domain Seven: Access to Care

Definition: *The individual's perceived physical availability of, and ready access to, healthcare services*

Question	Relevance to the domain 4=highly relevant 3=quite relevant 2=somewhat relevant 1=not relevant				Clarity of the question 4=clear 3=needs minor revisions 2=needs major revision 1=not clear			
	4	3	2	1	4	3	2	1
67. Where do you go to obtain care for yourself when you experience health problems or illness?	○	○	○	○	○	○	○	○
68. How easy is it for you to get to the clinic or hospital to be seen?	○	○	○	○	○	○	○	○
69. Who do you see when you need care for yourself?	○	○	○	○	○	○	○	○
70. How easy it is for you to get age-related routine or preventative health care (periodic checkups, immunizations, screening tests)	○	○	○	○	○	○	○	○
71. Are you able to easily get healthcare when needed for other family members who rely upon you?	○	○	○	○	○	○	○	○
72. What difficulties have you encountered in getting healthcare?	○	○	○	○	○	○	○	○
73. (For women of childbearing age), what difficulties have you encountered in obtaining health care in family planning or care throughout pregnancy?	○	○	○	○	○	○	○	○

Comments about the domain access to care:

Comments about the question items:

Domain Eight: Perceived Discrimination

Definition: *The individual's perceived prejudicial experiences of differential, marginal, or biased treatment, in seeking, accessing, and utilizing healthcare*

Question	Relevance to the domain 4=highly relevant 3=quite relevant 2=somewhat relevant 1=not relevant				Clarity of the question 4=clear 3=needs minor revisions 2=needs major revision 1=not clear			
	4	3	2	1	4	3	2	1
74. When you are ill, and seek help, are you provided with a timely appointment?	○	○	○	○	○	○	○	○
75. When you are ill, is there a lengthy delay in seeing your doctor or other healthcare provider?	○	○	○	○	○	○	○	○
76. Are you allowed with sufficient time to fully explain your problems to your doctor or other healthcare provider?	○	○	○	○	○	○	○	○
77. Do you feel that the doctor or other healthcare provider has an active interest in what you have to say?	○	○	○	○	○	○	○	○
78. Do you feel your problems are understood by your doctor or other healthcare provider?	○	○	○	○	○	○	○	○
79. Are you asked about your preferences for care?	○	○	○	○	○	○	○	○
80. Are your preferences for care followed?	○	○	○	○	○	○	○	○

Question	Relevance to the domain 4=highly relevant 3=quite relevant 2=somewhat relevant 1=not relevant				Clarity of the question 4=clear 3=needs minor revisions 2=needs major revision 1=not clear			
	4	3	2	1	4	3	2	1
81. Are you asked about self-care practices, including cultural practices, to alleviate illness?	○	○	○	○	○	○	○	○
82. When you have your appointment with the doctor or other healthcare provider, or undergo a procedure, or require hospitalization, are you treated with respect?	○	○	○	○	○	○	○	○
83. When you are experiencing severe pain or discomfort does the doctor or other healthcare provider take immediate action to alleviate this?	○	○	○	○	○	○	○	○

Domain Eight: Perceived Discrimination

Definition: *The individual's perceived prejudicial experiences of differential, marginal, or biased treatment, in seeking, accessing, and utilizing healthcare*

Question	Relevance to the domain 4=highly relevant 3=quite relevant 2=somewhat relevant 1=not relevant				Clarity of the question 4=clear 3=needs minor revisions 2=needs major revision 1=not clear			
	4	3	2	1	4	3	2	1
84. Are your questions concerning your care answered in a timely and satisfactory manner?	○	○	○	○	○	○	○	○
85. Are things explained to you in a manner that you can understand?	○	○	○	○	○	○	○	○
86. Are you provided with timely access to a certified medical interpreter when requested?	○	○	○	○	○	○	○	○

87. When it is medically advised to perform a treatment or medical procedure for health reasons are you explained the risks and benefits of this in a manner that you fully understand?

4	3	2	1	4	3	2	1
○	○	○	○	○	○	○	○

88. When you have questions concerning your care do the healthcare professional staff act on your behalf for your needs?

4	3	2	1	4	3	2	1
○	○	○	○	○	○	○	○

89. When you disagree with your care or treatments, does the doctor or other healthcare professional:

a. Listen attentively to your point of view?

4	3	2	1	4	3	2	1
○	○	○	○				

b. Communicate respectfully?

4	3	2	1	4	3	2	1
○	○	○	○				

c. Explore other treatment options and potential resultant outcomes?

4	3	2	1	4	3	2	1
○	○	○	○	○	○	○	○

d. Explain other treatment options and potential resultant outcomes in a manner that you understand?

4	3	2	1	4	3	2	1
○	○	○	○	○	○	○	○

Domain Eight: Perceived Discrimination

Definition: *The individual's perceived prejudicial experiences of differential, marginal, or biased treatment, in seeking, accessing, and utilizing healthcare*

Question	Relevance to the domain 4=highly relevant 3=quite relevant 2=somewhat relevant 1=not relevant				Clarity of the question 4=clear 3=needs minor revisions 2=needs major revision 1=not clear			
	4	3	2	1	4	3	2	1
90. Have you ever felt that your care was obstructed at any time when seeking care, or during your care, by any member of the healthcare team? Please describe.	○	○	○	○	○	○	○	○
91. Have you experienced discrimination at any time when seeking care, or during your care, by any member of the healthcare team? Please describe.	○	○	○	○	○	○	○	○

Comments about the domain perceived discrimination:

Comments about the question items:

Glossary

Displacement: The condition of persons who have been forced or obliged to flee or leave their homes or places of habitual residence to avoid the effects of armed conflict, generalized violence, violations of human rights, or natural or human-made disasters (IOM, 2019).

Immigration: The act of moving into another country, other than one's country of nationality or usual residence; the country of destination becomes the new country of usual residence (IOM, 2019).

International migrants: Persons who move away from their usual residence across an international border, either temporarily or permanently. Persons who are international migrants may include migrant workers, international students, humanitarian migrants, or persons moving for lifestyle or family reunification purposes (Batalova, 2022).

Migration: The movement of persons away from their place of usual residence, either across an international border or within a state (IOM, 2019).

Naturalization: Any mode of acquisition after birth of a nationality not previously held by the person, requiring an application by this person or his or her legal agent as well as an act

of granting nationality by a public authority (IOM, 2019).

Refugee: A person who is outside the country of their nationality, owing to a well-founded fear of persecution for reasons of race, religion, nationality, membership of a social group, or political opinion, and is unable or unwilling to avail themselves of the protection of that country, or owing to these fears is unable to return to it (IOM, 2019).

Relocation: Due to internal humanitarian emergencies, relocations are large-scale movements of civilians who face an immediate threat to life in a conflict setting to locations within the same country where they can be more effectively protected (IOM, 2019).

Repatriation: The personal right of a prisoner of war, civil detainee, refugee, or civilian to return to their country of nationality under specific conditions laid down in various international instruments (IOM, 2019).

Resettlement: Transfer of refugees from the country in which they have sought protection to another state that has agreed to admit them, as refugees, with permanent residence status (IOM, 2019).

References

Batalova, J. (2022). *Top statistics on global migration and migrants.* Migrant Policy Institute. https://www.migrationpolicy.org/article/top-statistics-global-migration-migrants

Catolico, O. (2013). Seeking life balance: The perceptions of health of Cambodian women in Resettlement. *The Journal of Transcultural Nursing, 24(3),* 236–245. https://doi.org/10.1177/1043659613481624

Clark, P. N., McFarland, M. R., Andrews, M. M., & Leininger, M. (2009). Caring: Some reflections on the impact of culture care theory by McFarland and Andrews and a conversation with Leininger. *Nursing Science Quarterly, 22(3)*, 233–239. https://doi.org/10.1177/0894318 409337020

Inter-Agency Standing Committee (IASC). (2019). *IASC Task Team on Inclusion of Disabilities in Humanitarian Action. Guidelines: Inclusion of persons with disabilities in humanitarian action.* https://interagencystandingcommittee.org/iasc-guidelines-on-inclusion-of-persons-with-disabilities-in-humanitarian-action-2019

Integral Human Development. (n.d.). Migratory profile: Mexico. https://migrants-refugees.va/resource-center/migratory-profiles/

International Organization for Migration (IOM). (2021). *World migration report 2022.* https://publications.iom.int/books/world-migration-report-2022

International Organization for Migration (IOM). (2024). *IOM strategic plan 2024–2028.* IOM Geneva.

Kleinman, A., Eisenberg, L., & Good, B. (1978). Culture, illness, and care: Clinical lessons from anthropologic and cross-cultural research. *Annals of Internal Medicine, 88(2)*, 251–258.

Leininger, M. M. (2006). Culture care diversity and universality theory and evolution of the ethnonursing method. In M. M. Leininger & M. R. McFarland (Eds.), *Culture care diversity and universality: A worldwide nursing theory* (2nd ed., pp. 1–41). Jones & Bartlett.

McGivern, V., Bluestone, K., & Lilly, D. (2020). *If not now, when? Keeping promises to older people affected by humanitarian crises.* HelpAge International. https://www.helpage.org/silo/files/if-not-now-when-report.pdf

Migration Policy Institute (MPI). (n.d.-a). *Age-sex pyramids of U.S. immigrant and native-born populations, 1970–present (Year: 2022).* https://www.migrationpolicy.org/programs/data-hub/charts/age-sex-pyramids-immigrant-and-native-born-population-over-time

Migration Policy Institute (MPI). (n.d.-b). *Top 25 destinations of international migrants (Year: 2020).* https://www.migrationpolicy.org/programs/data-hub/charts/top-25-destinations-international-migrants

Ruggles, S., Flood, S., Goeken, R., Schouweiler, M., & Sobek, M. (2022). *IPUMS USA: Version 12.0* [dataset]. IPUMS Center for Data Integration. https://doi.org/10.18128/D010.V12.0

United Nations. (n.d.). *International migrant stock 2020.* https://www.un.org/development/desa/pd/content/international-migrant-stock

United Nations. (2016). *Resolution adopted by the General Assembly on 19 September 2016: New York declaration for refugees and migrants.* https://www.un.org/en/development/desa/population/migration/generalassembly/docs/globalcompact/A_RES_71_1.pdf

United Nations. (2019). *Resolution adopted by the General Assembly on 19 December 2018: Global compact for safe, orderly and regular migration.* https://www.un.org/en/development/desa/population/migration/generalassembly/docs/globalcompact/A_RES_73_195.pdf

United Nations Office of the High Commissioner for Refugees (UNHCR). (n.d.). *About UNHCR.* https://www.unhcr.org/about-unhcr

United Nations Office of the High Commissioner for Refugees (UNHCR). (2023). *Global trends: Forced displacement in 2022.* https://www.unhcr.org/global-trends-report-2022

Ward, N., & Batalova, J. (2023). *Frequently requested statistics on immigrants and immigration to the United States.* Migration Policy Institute. https://www.migrationpolicy.org/sites/default/files/publications/frs-print-2023.pdf

World Bank. (2023). *World development report: Migrants, refugees, and societies.* https://www.worldbank.org/en/publication/wdr2023

World Health Organization (WHO). (2019a, May 23). *Promoting the health of refugees and migrants.* https://apps.who.int/gb/ebwha/pdf_files/WHA72/A72_25Rev1-en.pdf

World Health Organization (WHO). (2019b, October 2). *Refugee and migrant health at WHO: The new global action plan: Expectations, gaps, perspectives* [PowerPoint Slides]. Pan American Health Organization. https://www.paho.org/en/documents/presentation-refugee-and-migrant-health-who-new-global-action-plan-expectations-gaps

World Health Organization (WHO). (2022). *World report on the health of refugees and migrants.* https://www.who.int/publications/i/item/9789240054462

Selected Bibliography

Arola, A., Dahlin-Ivanoff, S., & Haggblom-Kronlof, G. (2020). Impact of a person-centred group intervention on life satisfaction and engagement in activities among persons in the context of migration. *Scandinavian Journal of Occupational Therapy, 27(4),* 269–279. https://doi.org/10.1080/11038128.2018.1515245

Arora, S., Bergland, A., Straiton, M., Rechel, B., & Debesay, J. (2018). Older migrants' access to healthcare: A thematic synthesis. *International Journal of Migration, Health and Social Care, 14(4),* 425–438. https://doi.org/10.1108/IJMHSC-05-2018-0032

Burns, S. D., Baker, E. H., Sheehan, C. M., & Markides, K. S. (2024). Disability among older immigrants in the United States: Exploring differences by region of origin and gender. *The International Journal of Aging and Human Development, 98(3),* 329–351. https://doi.org/10.1177/00914150231196093

Bustamante, L. H. U., Cerqueira, R. O., Leclerc, E., & Brietzke, E. (2018). Stress, trauma, and posttraumatic stress disorder in migrants: A comprehensive review. *Brazilian Journal of Psychiatry, 40,* 220–225. https://doi.org/10.1590/1516-4446-2017-2290

Climate Migration 101 https://www.migrationpolicy.org/article/climate-migration-101-explainer

Dominguez-Mujica, J., & Rodriguez-Rodriguez, M.A. (2023). Older adult Cubans moving to the Canary Islands (Spain): Migrant strategies in later life. *Journal of Aging Studies, 64,* 1–7. https://doi.org/10.1016./j.jaging.2022.101098.

Georgeou, N., Schismenos, S., Wali, N., Mackay, K., & Moraitakis, E. (2021). A scoping review of aging experiences among culturally and linguistically diverse people in Australia: Toward better aging policy and cultural well-being for migrant and refugee adults. *The Gerontologist, 63(1),* 182–199. https://doi.org/10.1093/geront/gnab191

Hawkins, M. M., Holliday, D. D., Weinhardt, L. S., Florsheim, P., Ngui, E., & AbuZahra, T. (2022). *BMC Public Health, 22*(755), 1–17. https://doi.org/10.1186/s12889-022-13042-x

Irving, J. (2024). *"I go to sleep on an empty stomach": Improving the inclusion of older people in humanitarian nutrition planning and response.* HelpAge International. https://www.helpage.org/wp-content/uploads/2024/03/I-sleep-on-an-empty-stomach.pdf

Jung, Y. M. (2022). Pathways of aging in migration and their association with the quality of life. *Asian and Pacific Migration Journal, 31(2),* 99–117. https://doi.org/10.1177/01171968221109038

Kadowaki, L., Koehn, S. D., Brotman, S., Simard, J., Ferrer, I., Raymond, E., & Orzeck, P. (2023). Learning from the lived experiences of aging immigrants: Extending the reach of photovoice using world café methods. *Journal of Community Engagement and Scholarship, 16*(1), 1–18.

Kaplan, J., Lazarescou, N., Huang, S., Ali, S., Banu, S., Du, Y. B., & Shrestha, S. (2021). Overview of challenges faced by refugees following resettlement in Houston, Texas: A qualitative study at five refugee resettlement agencies. *International Journal of Migration, Health and Social Care, 18*(1), 1–15. https://doi.org/10.1108/IJMHSC-01-2021-0009

Lee, S. (2024). Social exclusion of U.S. immigrants in the 21st century: A systematic review of qualitative studies. *International Social Work, 67(1),* 194–207. https://doi.org/10.1177/00208728221087045

Maleku, A., Espana, M., Jarrott, S., Karandikar, S., & Parekh, R. (2022). We are aging too! Exploring the social impact of late-life migration among older immigrants in the United States. *Journal of Immigrant and Refugee Studies, 20(3),* 365–382. https://doi.org//10.1080/15562948.2021.1929643

Raad, I. I., Chaftari, A.-M., Dib, R. W., Graviss, E. A., & Hachem, R. (2018). Emerging outbreaks associated with conflict and failing healthcare systems in the Middle East. *Infection Control & Hospital Epidemiology, 39,* 1230–1236. https://doi.org/10.1017/ice.2018.177

Siddiq, H., Ajrouch, K., Elhaija, A., Kayali, N., & Heilemann, M. (2023). Addressing the mental health needs of older adult refugees: Perspectives of multi-sector community key informants. *SSM-Qualitative Research in Health, 3,* 1–9. https://doi.org/10.1016/m.ssmqr.2023.100269

Siddiq, H., Alemi, Q., & Lee, E. (2023). A qualitative inquiry of older Afghan refugee women's individual and sociocultural factors of health and health care experiences in the United States. *The Journal of Transcultural Nursing, 34(2),* 143–150. https://doi.org/10.1177/10436596221149692

Websites

Center for Migration Studies (CMS) of New York https://cmsny.org/about/initiatives/catholic-immigrant-integration-initiative/

Data: Estimates of the US Undocumented and Other Immigrant Populations https://cmsny.org/research-and-policy/data/

Climate Change and Migration: Special Issue https://www.migrationpolicy.org/programs/migration-information-source/special-issue-climate-change-and-migration

CLIMB Database https://migrationnetwork.un.org/climb

International Organization for Migration https://www.iom.int/

IOM Interactive Migration Data Portal

Migration and Human Mobility: Key Global Figures, November, 2023 https://www.migrationdataportal.org/resource/key-global-migration-figures

Migration Data Portal https://www.migrationdataportal.org/

Migration Policy Institute Regions: https://www.migrationpolicy.org/regions/africa-sub-saharan

Migration Policy Institute State Immigration Profiles: United States

Demographics and Social https://www.migrationpolicy.org/data/state-profiles/state/demographics/US

English Proficiency

https://www.migrationpolicy.org/data/state-profiles/state/language/US#

Workforce All Indicators https://www.migrationpolicy.org/data/state-profiles/state/workforce/US#

Income and Poverty

https://www.migrationpolicy.org/data/state-profiles/state/income/US#

Age Sex Pyramids https://www.migrationpolicy.org/programs/data-hub/charts/age-sex-pyramids-immigrant-and-native-born-population-over-time

United Nations Department of Economic and Social Affairs Statistics Division SDG Indicators Database, UN SDG Data Portal https://unstats.un.org/sdgs/dataportal

United Nations Population Division

https://www.un.org/development/desa/pd/data/global-migration-database

https://www.un.org/development/desa/pd/content/international-migrant-stock

United Nations Department of Economic and Social Affairs Statistics Division (2023).

Demographic Yearbook, 2022, 73rd Issue https://unstats.un.org/unsd/demographic-social/products/dyb/index.cshtml

Demographic and Social Statistics, International Migration https://unstats.un.org/unsd/demographic-social/sconcerns/migration/

Demographic and Social Statistics, Gender Statistics https://worlds-women-2020-data-undesa.hub.arcgis.com/

Evidence and Data for Gender Equality https://unstats.un.org/edge

Country Profiles: USA https://unstats.un.org/sdgs/dataportal/countryprofiles/usa

UN SDG Report 2023 https://unstats.un.org/sdgs/report/2023/

UNHCR Global Trends Report, 2022 https://www.unhcr.org/sites/default/files/2023-06/global-trends-report-2022.pdf

Reports and Briefs

HelpAge International https://helpageusa.org/

Adem, J. M., Anshiso, D., Kebede, K., & Alamerie, K. (2023). *Enhancing financial inclusion of older urban poor in Ethiopia: A call for action.* HelpAge International. https://www.helpage.org/wp-content/uploads/2023/11/Enhancing-financial-inclusion-of-older-urban-poor-in-Ethiopia.pdf

Banks, N., & Storey, K. (2024). *Roles Reimagined: Stories of Challenges and Self-Reliance from Older People in Northwest Syria.* HelpAge International. https://www.helpage.org/wp-content/uploads/2024/02/Roles-Reimagined.pdf

Charveriat, C., Bodin, E., Cartier, B., & Haq, G. (2023). *Climate justice in an ageing world: Discussion paper.* HelpAge International. https://www.helpage.org/wp-content/uploads/2023/11/Climate-justice-in-an-ageing-world.pdf

Foiadelli, F., Patel, T., Petitprez, J., & Horstead, K. (2024). *Advancing gender equality through social protection in an ageing world: A call for action.* HelpAge International. https://www.helpage.org/wp-content/uploads/2024/03/Gender-Equality-Briefing.pdf

Galvani, F., & Chandranshu. (2022). *Towards a social pension for all older people in the Occupied Palestinian Territory.* HelpAge International. https://www.helpage.org/wp-content/uploads/2023/07/Towards-a-social-pension-for-all-older-people-in-the-Occupied-Palestinian-Territory-ENG-2.pdf

Gascón, S., & Saieg, M. (2023). *Impact of the economic and social crisis on older people in Argentina.* HelpAge International. https://www.helpage.org/wp-content/uploads/2023/09/Argentina-Addressing-the-food-fuel-and-finance-crisis-Policy-brief.pdf

HelpAge Global Network. (2024). *Statement for the 68th Session of the United Nations Commission on the Status of Women (CSW 68), March 2024.* https://www.helpage.org/wp-content/uploads/2023/10/Statement-for-CSW68.pdf

HelpAge International. (2023). *Lessons learned 2022/23.* https://www.helpage.org/wp-content/uploads/2023/10/Learning-202223-Online.pdf

HelpAge International. (2024). *A lifetime of suffering: The challenges faced by older people in Gaza.* https://www.helpage.org/wp-content/uploads/2024/02/Gaza-Briefing-.pdf

Shoujaa, K., Hijazi, S., & El Zayed, M. (2023). *Older people in crisis in Lebanon: An urgent need for action*. HelpAge International. https://www.helpage.org/wp-content/uploads/2023/05/Food-Fuel-Finance-crisis_Policy-brief-Lebanon.pdf

Suriastini, N. W., Sabdono, E. A. J., Herawati, F., Asanti, E., & Ambarwati, T. P. (2023). *Examining decent work in Indonesia: Experiences of older rural women entrepreneurs in Central Java*. HelpAge International. https://www.helpage.org/wp-content/uploads/2023/10/Examining-decent-work-in-Indonesia.pdf

Williamson, C. (2022). *Achieving Universal Health Coverage fit for an ageing world*. HelpAge International. https://helpageusa.org/wp-content/uploads/2023/06/Universal-Health-Coverage-Report_FINAL.pdf

Williamson, C., & De Pauw, M. (2023). *Healthy ageing for us all: What older people say about their right to health*. HelpAge International. https://helpageusa.org/wp-content/uploads/2024/01/healthy-ageing-report.pdf

Woroniecka-Krzyżanowska, D., & Urbańska, B. *"Everyone has their own story, but it hurts us all the same": Learning from the experiences of older Ukrainian refugees in Poland*. HelpAge International. https://www.helpage.org/wp-content/uploads/2023/09/We-all-have-our-own-story-ENGLISH.pdf

Websites

WELLNESS AND QUALITY OF LIFE IN AGING

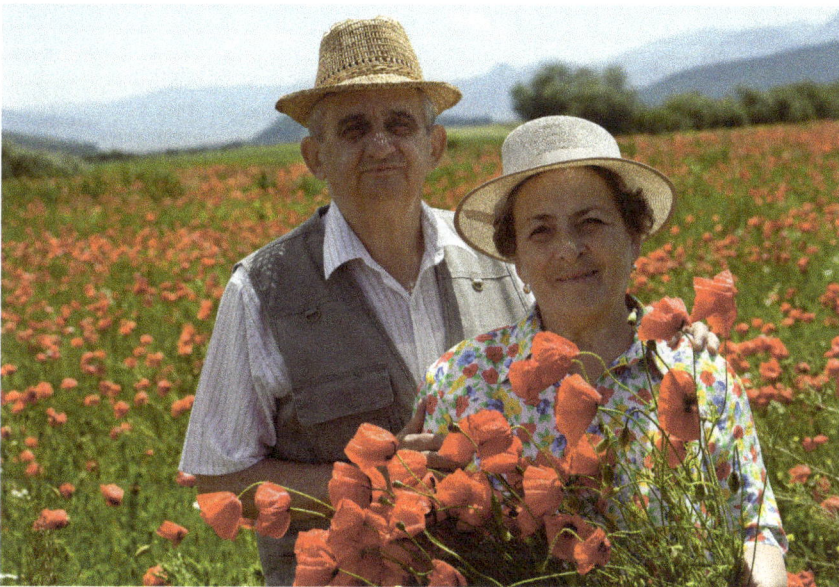

Image 7.1

Overview

The literature is replete with information that sufficiently addresses the physical aspects of aging, diseases, and chronic illness. It is not the intent of this chapter to replicate that information. Rather, this chapter focuses on supporting the older adult in health promotion and quality of life even in the presence of chronic illness. This chapter emphasizes concepts useful in maintaining states of wellness, preventing illness, and managing chronic illness. These main concepts are pain and comfort, thermoregulation, immunity, skin integrity, mobility, oxygenation and perfusion, sleep, and resilience (stress and coping). This chapter also introduces interprofessional collaboration in assisting the older adult to maintain wellness and quality of life.

Outcomes

The learner:

1. Utilizes evidence-based assessments in planning care with the older adult

2. Establishes mutual goals of care in an atmosphere of trust and respect based on values, preferences, and capabilities of the older adult

3. Utilizes opportunities at the point of care to teach the older adult (and their caregiver/family) about health promotion and self-care actions to maintain wellness, prevent illness, and/or manage chronic illness

4. Collaborates effectively with the interprofessional team to facilitate the achievement of mutual goals

Introduction

The science and knowledge about aging continue to evolve. The knowledge available aids in understanding, planning care, and helping ensure that older adults age successfully in place within their communities. Study of the aging process and the science of aging has led to theories of aging from various perspectives—the biological-physiological and psychosocial-emotional perspectives.

Biological-Physiological Changes and the Aging Process

Cellular changes that occur with aging are different for each individual. However, the ability of cells to reproduce decreases over time. Internal contributing factors to cellular aging include inflammation from various sources, including emotional stress, and lifestyle choices, such as smoking and substance use. The environment and external factors also have a role in cellular aging. Examples of these factors are secondhand cigarette smoke, pollution smog and ozone, pesticides, and radiation.

From the biological-physiological point of view, it is thought that portions of the DNA found in chromosomes, or telomeres, play a role in the aging process. Telomere length is thought to be an indicator of physiological age. As cells reproduce, telomeres shorten. This shortening leads to cellular aging and ultimately cellular death.

Neurocognitive

Cognition is the ability to acquire, store, and use information. It involves language, memory, and executive function. Research and information has focused on cognitive decline and progressive deteriorating disease states such as dementia and Alzheimer's disease. Emerging research has emphasized cognitive function, intellectual capacity, and performance, which are mediated by the interplay of multiple factors such as nutrition, physical function, life experience, environmental changes, smoking, alcohol, and education. In an aging neurological system, processing complex and increased amounts of information takes more time, and this is not the result of a disease state. Cognitive abilities remain intact, with normal declines that occur with aging, such as verbal fluency, naming of objects, and visuospatial abilities.

Cognitive reserve applies to brain health. It stems from the concept of neuroplasticity, in which the strength and complexity of neuronal connections allows for information and cognition to emerge. Therefore, stimulating the brain increases tissue formation, enhances synaptic connections, and improves cognitive reserve. Sleep also plays a role in promoting learning-dependent synapse formation. Cognitive reserve and new capacities in later adulthood can be developed through challenging cognitive and sensorimotor activities and meaningful interactions.

Cardiovascular

Much of the research evidence focuses on cardiac disease states, and this is well documented in the research literature. However, there is little mention about the normal changes that occur in an aging cardiovascular system without underlying disease. Normal cardiovascular changes are loss of elasticity and stiffening of the vessels within the circulatory system. The heart is a muscle and functions as a pump. With advancing age, there is stiffening of the left ventricle with little change in ejection fraction, or left ventricular output. There is little decrease in resting heart rate, but there is a decrease in maximum heart rate in response to exertion and stressors. The target maximum heart rate is calculated as "220 minus age." B-type natriuretic peptide, or brain natriuretic peptide, a protein hormone (BNP), increases with age in healthy older adults. BNP helps regulate circulation by widening or dilating blood vessels and by excreting water and sodium through the kidneys.

An aging cardiovascular system places the older adult at risk for cardiac diseases such as hypertension, heart failure, myocardial infarction, angina, and stroke. Persons may experience cardiac dysrhythmias such as atrial fibrillation, which may be caused by underlying disease. Preventive early screening and teaching persons how to stay healthy and how to prevent complications in the presence of disease can contribute to successful aging in place. Blood pressure screening, monitoring, periodic physical assessment with diagnostic lab work, and lifestyle changes can mitigate risks and prevent further complications in disease states. Nutrition (low sodium, low saturated fat, and low cholesterol foods), physical activity, and smoking and alcohol cessation are ways of self-management.

Respiratory

Normal age-related changes in the respiratory system are loss of chest wall elasticity, or compliance, and decreased functional reserves. Functional reserves are the lung capacities, which are vital capacity and total lung capacity. Vital capacity is the inspiratory reserve volume, tidal volume, and expiratory reserve volume, which is the maximum amount of air one can expel from the lungs after filling the lungs to their maximum extent and expiring to the maximum extent (4,600 milliliters). The total lung capacity is the maximum volume to which the lungs can be expanded with the greatest possible inspiratory effort (5,800 milliliters). Normal ventilation is accomplished by the muscles of inspiration, which are the diaphragm and the intercostal muscles. At rest in the young adult, this is about 2,300 milliliters. These volumes are important, as they affect alveolar ventilation. Alveoli are the tiny air sacs at the end of the respiratory tree where gas exchange and perfusion occur.

Changes in the respiratory system with age place the older adult at risk for compromised ventilation and gas exchange. Factors contributing to this compromise are underlying illnesses such as an acquired bacterial infection resulting in pneumonia, chronic obstructive pulmonary disease (COPD), an inflammatory response to a virus, or an allergic reaction. Smoking, exposure to secondary smoke, environmental air quality, air pollutants, and allergens are also triggers for compromised lung function.

Exercise helps promote gas exchange, and avoidance of illness decreases the risk of poor lung function. Older persons can monitor air quality, environmental allergens, and pollutants prior to outdoor exercise.

Gastrointestinal

Multiple age-related changes occur within the gastrointestinal (GI) system. The GI system includes the mouth, esophagus, stomach, small intestines, and the accessory organs, liver and gallbladder. Age-related changes are the wear and tear of the teeth with loss of enamel and dentin; gum recession; slowed peristalsis, decreased gastric motility; decline in hydrochloric acid production and intrinsic factor necessary for vitamin B12 utilization; decreased intestinal peristalsis; and changes in epithelial membranes (mucosal lining), villi, and vascular perfusion. There are no specific normal age-related changes to the liver and gallbladder.

Older persons may be prone to dental caries and gum disease and digestive discomfort. More importantly, absorption of important nutrients such as lipids, amino acids, glucose, calcium, and iron are affected. Dental caries and gum disease can be mitigated through good oral health care, preventive screening, assessments, and treatment. Additional health promotion measures are the maintenance of adequate hydration, nutrition, and activity. Contrary to popular belief, constipation is not a normal part of aging. It is often due to medication side effects, immobility, and life habits.

Musculoskeletal

Structures affected by age-related changes in the musculoskeletal system are dryer ligaments, tendons, and joints; decreased muscle mass; reduced bone mineral density; and decreased body water. Intervertebral discs become thin as a result of gravity and dehydration, resulting in a shortened or stooped appearance (kyphosis) as a result of reduced bone mineral density. Consequently, persons experience reduced flexibility and reduced strength. Additionally, there is an increased risk of spontaneous and traumatic fractures, and an increased risk of dehydration.

Musculoskeletal changes place the older adult at risk for osteoporosis, fractures, and arthritis. Risks can be minimized throughout life by consuming a calcium-rich diet with vitamin D, maintaining a healthy body weight, and maintaining strength and flexibility through weight-bearing exercise.

Renal

The renal system regulates fluid and electrolytes in the body, thereby maintaining acid–base balance. The structure responsible for this function is the glomerulus, which is a network of capillaries. The glomerulus filters out excess ions and unwanted substances into the urine and retains or reabsorbs back into the bloodstream wanted substances such as water and electrolytes. The glomerular filtration rate (GFR), or the rate at which the glomerulus filters blood flow through the kidneys, is about 1,200 milliliters/minute in young adults. As persons age, the GFR decreases approximately 10% per decade, or to about 600 milliliters/minute in an 80-year-old. Even with this change the body is able to maintain daily homeostasis.

Older adults have a decreased reserve capacity to handle fluid overloads or deficits and are at risk for renal failure. These risks can be mitigated by teaching the older persons the effects of prescribed medications that impact kidney function and about invasive diagnostic tests where contrast media may be used, which could affect renal function. Maintaining adequate fluid intake, balanced nutrition, and knowledge of substances contained in foods and food additives are health-promotional strategies to influence the older adult's informed choices.

Integumentary

Age-related changes in skin include dryness, thinning, reduced melanocytes, decreased elasticity, decreased sebum production, and increased time needed for cell renewal. Consequently, older persons may be at risk for solar damage, bruises, and skin tears. A cut or laceration may take longer to heal and predispose the individual to infections. The older person may experience reduced ability to withstand cooler or hotter changes in environmental temperatures.

Avoidance of injury, protection from ultraviolet sunlight (ultraviolet protection factor [UPF] clothing, hat, sunglasses, and sunblock), hydration, use of skin moisturizers, and nutrition are ways to maintain healthy skin. Research evidence indicates that nutrients for healthy skin include vitamin A, vitamin B complex, vitamin C, vitamin D, vitamin E, biotin, and minerals (chromium, iron, selenium, and zinc). Regular assessments and skin checkups from a health professional are also preventive strategies.

Sensory

Presbyopia, a normal age-related change in near vision, occurs around midlife. Reduced responsiveness of the pupils and changes in the lens are responsible for difficulty in accommodation to lighting. Eyeglasses, magnifying glasses, and other optical devices may be needed for close work or reading. High-intensity lighting on an object or surface may help with decreased accommodation to various levels of lighting. Sunglasses offer protection from ultraviolet sunlight and help reduce glare. Routine assessment by an eye care professional is essential. Visual acuity testing, measurement of intraocular pressures, and funduscopic examination are necessary for early detection of changes and appropriate intervention. Nutrition to promote healthy eyes includes leafy green vegetables and fish. Additional health promotion strategies are avoidance of cigarette smoking and maintaining blood pressure within normal limits.

Presbycusis, the loss of the ability to hear high-frequency sounds, also occurs with advancing age. This may be mitigated by reducing environmental noise and allowing the older adult time to decipher or process what is being said. As with vision changes in later life, routine professional assessment and evaluation of sensorineural hearing loss is imperative. Strategies to promote healthy hearing include avoidance of exposure to excessive loud noise, smoking cessation, nutrition, and blood pressure control.

Immune System

With advancing age, normal changes are decreased immunity and a delayed immune response. Consequently, older persons are at risk for increased infections and decreased signs and symptoms of illness as compared to that seen in younger adults. Normal core temperatures of older adults range from 95 to 97 degrees Fahrenheit, with an average of 96 degrees Fahrenheit. Therefore, a temperature of 99 degrees Fahrenheit, which would signal a low-grade fever in a younger adult, may indicate serious illness in an older adult. Careful assessments of any change in basal temperature in conjunction with cognitive assessments or injuries are imperative.

Concepts Related to Biological-Physiological Processes of Aging

Central to wellness in older persons are concepts of safety and risk reduction. These concepts are embodied in the Quality and Safety Education for Nurses (QSEN) competencies. The QSEN competencies define knowledge, skills, and attitudes for safe practice across six domains: (1) patient-centered care, (2) teamwork and collaboration, (3) evidence-based practice (EBP), (4) quality improvement (QI), (5) safety, and (6) informatics (QSEN, n.d.). The competencies can be used to determine the quality and extent to which individual health care professionals, teams, and organizations integrate safety and risk reduction in older adult wellness and care.

Concepts of health promotion and health maintenance in older persons are pain management and comfort, thermoregulation, immunity, skin integrity, mobility, oxygenation and perfusion, intracranial regulation, sleep, and resilience (stress management and coping).

Pain Management and Comfort

A myth of aging is that older persons are expected to experience pain or that pain is a normal part of aging. Pain is not a normal age-related change; its presence signifies underlying disease, disease progression, or a complication of illness and/or treatment. Pain is a complex, subjective, and personal phenomenon influenced by cultural, bio-psycho-social, and environmental factors. Determining what pain means to the older person, their measures taken to alleviate it, and a comprehensive review of bio-psycho-social systems are important assessments. Whether pain is acute or chronic, a goal of care is to provide comfort to maintain optimum function and well-being. The presence of pain is often pervasive and affects nutrition, mobility and function, circulation, cognition, and rest.

Evidence-based tools have been developed for pain assessment (see Appendix B). The Pain Assessment in Advanced Dementia (PAINAD), the Pain Assessment Checklist for Seniors with Limited Ability to Communicate (PACSLAC-II), and the Facies Pain Scale-Revised (FPS-R) can be used in assessing pain in older persons who are unable to communicate or express their pain through language.

It should be noted that older persons have individual needs, tolerances, and responses to pain medication. Beer's criteria are useful in assessing and determining pain management needs. Beer's criteria identify potentially inappropriate medications for older persons, and the risks of use must be carefully weighed against the benefits. These criteria are updated about every 5 years by a panel of experts of the American Geriatrics Society (American Geriatrics Society Beers Criteria Update Panel, 2023).

Thermoregulation

Older adults experience fluctuations in maintaining core body temperature in climate extremes. The ability of the body to increase heat production in extreme cold or to facilitate heat loss in extreme heat is influenced by a number of factors—cognitive impairment, preexisting medical conditions (hypothyroidism or hyperthyroidism, for example), nutrition, and hydration status. Important assessments include vital signs, physical assessment, environmental assessment, and identification of community and emergency resources during weather extremes.

Protective measures during cold weather extremes that can be utilized by older adults are the use of warm, dry clothing that can be layered, warm blankets, head coverings, and adequate ambient temperature. Physical activity also helps generates body heat. Wind drafts at doors and windows can be minimized using insulating curtains. During extreme hot weather, opening windows and the use of fans, especially during cooler periods, can help maintain ambient temperature in the absence of home air-conditioning. Public buildings, libraries, and shopping malls are also places where temperatures are regulated. Communities may advertise "cooling centers" where people can go for respite from outdoor heat. These centers may be located through city or county websites and directories. Physical exertion should be limited during extreme heat to minimize the risk of hyperthermia. Hydration, cool water baths, cooling towels placed around the neck, appropriate lightweight clothing, and shelter from the heat are strategies to maintain normal body temperature.

Local city, community, and county websites may provide vital information for older adults to prepare for environmental extremes in temperature and natural disasters. Natural disasters affect food and water supply, shelter, public utilities, transportation, communication systems, and access to health care. Strategies for health maintenance are education, safety precautions, preparation, and ready supplies, including medications and first aid supplies, for unexpected or unprecedented events.

Immunity

The immune system staves off harmful microorganisms, removes dead or damaged cells, and recognizes and removes abnormal cells. These functions diminish with age due to decreased lymphocyte functions of special cells—T lymphocytes and B lymphocytes. T cells destroy infected and cancerous cells; B cells produce antibodies to fight infection. Older persons should be assessed for chronic conditions that may contribute to a compromised immune system: human immunodeficiency virus (HIV), malnutrition, cancer, chronic obstructive pulmonary disease (COPD), asthma, and autoimmune diseases (fibromyalgia, multiple sclerosis, lupus erythematosus, allergies). Medical and pharmacological treatments for chronic conditions also suppress the immune response. High-risk behaviors, substance abuse, and excessive alcohol abuse lead to compromised immunity and risk for infection.

Wellness promotion strategies to boost immunity are a nutritious diet, hydration, exercise, avoidance of high-risk behaviors and use of substances, decreased exposure to environmental triggers, and avoidance of others who are infectious. Important strategies for health maintenance are vaccinations recommended by the Centers for Disease Control (CDC). Among these recommended vaccinations are influenza, COVID-19, pneumovax, shingles, tetanus, hepatitis, and periodic boosters. Evidence-based information and education provided to older adults facilitate informed decision-making. Refusal of vaccines or vaccine hesitancy, whether based on myth or religious or cultural beliefs, can be explored in a tactful, respectful manner. Individuals may need time to reflect on their personal choices, the potential consequences, and their decisions to follow through or not follow through with vaccinations. Nonetheless, giving the older adult a means of direct, immediate contact and communication with the health care provider for more information, and/or when they are ready to receive vaccinations, is helpful.

Skin Integrity

Skin integrity is the structurally intact and physiologically functioning epithelial tissues (epidermis, dermis, subcutaneous) and mucous membranes. The skin is an extensive protective organ. Skin changes are the result of decreased thickness, loss of moisture, elasticity, and decreased circulation. Disruptions to skin integrity are associated with sun exposure and environmental damage, poor perfusion, exposure to chemical irritants, radiation, exposure to extremes in temperature, ulcerations, medical treatments (including medications), and invasive surgical procedures. Poor nutrition and hydration, decreased mobility, and immunosuppression contribute to impaired skin integrity. A thorough history, assessment, and examination of skin surfaces, oral mucosa, conjunctiva, and sclera are important.

General skin hygiene, bathing, and use of moisturizers help maintain skin integrity. Health and wellness strategies include measures such as adequate nutrition and hydration, physical activity, avoidance of overexposure to ultraviolet sun rays, and avoidance or protection from irritants. Chronic conditions such as diabetes can affect skin circulation, perfusion, and wound healing. Older adults can be taught to inspect their skin regularly for changes, signs of infection, and poor wound healing, and to seek professional help for additional screening, monitoring, and care. Older adults should also be informed of skin-related medication side effects and also how to report them and seek professional help.

Mobility

Mobility is purposeful movement and involves coordination of the musculoskeletal, nervous, and circulatory systems. Mobility is associated with one's independence. Factors affecting mobility include pain and acute or chronic illnesses affecting bones, joints, muscles, the central nervous system, and the circulatory and respiratory systems. Mobility assessment includes a complete health and social history. Attention to balance, fatigue, falls, and activities of daily living are important. Important and useful evidence-based assessments include those related to functional mobility, activities of daily living, and instrumental activities of daily living (IADL). Examples of these assessments are the Katz Index of Independence in Activities of Daily Living (ADL), Fall Risk Assessment for Adults: The Hendrich II Fall Risk Model, and the Lawton Instrumental Activities of Daily Living (IADL) Scale (Hartford Institute for Geriatric Nursing [HIGN], n.d.).

Strategies for wellness in mobility are regular physical activity at the highest level possible, optimum nutrition with adequate calcium and protein, maintenance of a healthy body weight, and maintenance of environmental safety. Providing education about the proper use of adaptive equipment and other mobility aids is essential to safety and the prevention of injuries in older persons. Examples of equipment include canes, wheelchairs, walkers, lifts, prosthetics, and other assistive technology devices. Equipment should be adjusted to suit the needs and preferences of the older adult, with attention to safety. The home environment should also be assessed for safe use of adaptive devices and injury prevention.

Perfusion and Oxygenation

Perfusion is blood flow through the arteries and capillaries, which delivers oxygen and nutrients and removes cellular waste. Decreased elasticity of the vascular system, stenosis of heart valves, and atherosclerosis contribute to altered perfusion and oxygenation. Modifiable risk factors are smoking, increased serum lipids, inactivity or sedentary lifestyle, obesity, diabetes, and hypertension. A comprehensive health history and physical assessment, including episodes of pain, edema (swelling), dizziness or fainting, and dyspnea (shortness of breath) are essential. Routine screening and diagnostic tests may include blood tests (complete blood count, electrolytes, cardiac enzymes, and serum lipids), a 12-lead electrocardiogram (EKG), an exercise cardiac stress test, and a chest X-ray.

Older persons can be provided information, education, and resources for reducing modifiable risk factors. A healthy diet, regular exercise, and blood pressure maintenance within normal limits are strategies for wellness. While there are many over-the-counter devices available for home use, older adults should be informed about their proper use and technique, calibration, conditions under which readings are taken (resting blood pressure), and interpretation of results. This information should also be shared with a health care professional or primary care provider.

Intracranial Regulation

Intracranial regulation refers to the mechanisms or conditions that affect intracranial processing and functioning. Structures involved in regulating compliance and balance for optimal brain functioning are the skull, brain, meninges, circulatory system, and cerebrospinal fluid. As with other concepts related to homeostasis, a thorough history and physical examination of the older adult is important. Inquiries of the older person include the presence of the following: numbness; paralysis; loss of consciousness; changes in memory; changes in vision, hearing, speech, balance, or gait; difficulty chewing or swallowing; headache; vomiting; and head injuries.

Testing of the cranial nerves is an important part of the neurological assessment. Evidence-based tools for assessment of mental status and neurological function include the Mini Mental Status exam, the Glasgow Coma Scale (GCS), the Mental Status Assessment of Older Adults: The Mini-Cog, and the Montreal Cognitive Assessment (MoCA). The reliability and validity of these assessment tools are documented in the research literature. It should be noted, however, that a single assessment test administered at a single point in time may not be an accurate indicator of the older person's brain functioning. Close observations and assessments administered consistently over time, in conjunction with other diagnostic tests and assessments of functioning, can provide more accurate information. Optimum brain health is supported through the lifestyle choices mentioned throughout this chapter—smoking cessation, maintaining a healthy weight, and regular physical exercise. Healthy lifestyle choices reduce the risk of vascular disease and stroke. Effective management of chronic illnesses, such as diabetes, hypertension, and chronic obstructive pulmonary disease, also helps optimize brain health.

Older adults who have had a stroke can successfully recover and regain function through rehabilitation. The Stroke Scale developed by the National Institutes of Health can be used by health care providers to assess neurological function (National Institute of Neurological Disorders and Stroke, n.d.).

Sleep and Rest

Sleep and adequate rest are often overlooked. Sleep is a basic need and restores mental and physical function. Multiple factors affect sleep: physiological (changes in circadian rhythm, chronic illness, pain, medications, lack of exercise), psychological (stressors, anxiety, loss), and environmental (noises, different environment, caregiving for older adult dependent). Sleep deprivation affects learning and memory and has been associated with road and workplace safety hazards. In addition to decreased function, there is evidence that sleep deficiency is linked to a number of health problems (heart disease, hypertension, stroke, diabetes, obesity, cancer, and decreased immune response), poor health outcomes, and premature mortality.

Sleep disorders that affect older adults are insomnia and sleep apnea. Insomnia is difficulty falling asleep and staying asleep (sleep initiation, duration, consolidation) that results in daytime impairment and is persistent at least three times a week for at least one month. In the case of sleep apnea, breathing repeatedly stops and starts. This disorder may be due to problems in the central nervous system or to an upper airway obstruction.

Sleep problems should be thoroughly investigated. While medications can be prescribed to help induce sleep, their use should be short-term. Benzodiazepines (depressants) or other sedative hypnotics have detrimental side effects such as changes in mental status (delirium, memory loss) and increased risk for falls, fractures, and motor vehicle accidents. Over-the-counter sleep aid preparations often contain ingredients that are not regulated and their efficacy is unknown. Sleep apnea can be managed with lifestyle changes and the use of breathing devices (continuous positive airway pressure device, or CPAP).

A number of nonpharmacological strategies help promote sleep hygiene: regular exercise and a healthy diet, a consistent sleep schedule, a quiet and relaxing room at a comfortable temperature, limiting bright light exposure, avoidance of caffeine and alcohol, and relaxation techniques.

Psychosocial-Emotional Aspects of Aging: Stress, Coping and Adaptation, and Resilience

The previous section focused on biological and physiological aspects of aging and strategies for health promotion and wellness. A whole-person approach to aging is inclusive of the psychosocial and emotional aspects of aging. There is much in the literature that examines these aspects of aging. This section focuses on the stress response, coping and adaptation, and resilience. Strategies for healthy aging in the psychosocial-emotional realms are identified. It is appropriate to discuss the stress response, as older adults have likely encountered multiple stressors in their lifetime. Older persons are unique, and responses to stressors are also personal and individual.

Stress and Eustress

Stress is an event or demand (physiological, environmental, or psychosocial) that an individual perceives, appraises, and determines whether such an event or demand is challenging or threatening, and whether resources are available to meet the event or demand. Physiologically, the body responds to stress through the production of glucocorticoid to maintain homeostasis. This response is accomplished through the neuroendocrine system, or HPA(hypothalamus-pituitary-adrenal)-axis regulation. In short, the hypothalamus stimulates the anterior pituitary gland to produce adrenocorticotropic hormone (ACTH); ACTH in turn stimulates the adrenal cortex to secrete glucocorticoids. This mechanism is effective for short-term stress. In chronic stress states, the HPA-axis becomes unresponsive. Exhaustion results in a chronic stress state, and persons become susceptible to other illnesses. Eustress, on the other hand, is defined as a positive form of stress, in which an event or demand causes physiological and cognitive changes that are beneficial to health, well-being, motivation, and performance.

Stressors or life events, experiences, and situations may induce the stress response in older persons. Examples of stressors are:

- Loss of network: partner or spouse, family members, relatives, friends, other relationships with people who constitute a significant social support network, such as fictive kin

- Change in socioeconomic status: loss of employment or change in employment, financial instability, decrease or loss of income, accumulation of debt

- Change in functional ability: inability to manage self-care for acute or chronic illness, level of independence, lack of transportation, or inability to drive

- Increased caregiving responsibilities: primary caregiver for dependent partner, spouse; primary parenting responsibilities for grandchildren in the absence of biological parents

- Occurrence of multiple events or demands all at once, or within a brief span of time

- Repeated messages and attitudes of ageism (stigma, bias, and discrimination) toward older adults from multiple sources at the individual, social, and institutional levels. Health care providers, family, public media and news outlets, and other agencies within the community (ex: banks, insurance agencies, auto services, housing agencies, public services/transportation, utility companies) are examples of systems through which ageist attitudes are perpetuated.

An inability to meet basic needs and costs of living, potential risk for isolation, rapid health deterioration, unmet self-actualization needs, and perceptions of decreased self-worth and self-esteem are all consequences of stressors. Older adults are denied basic rights and are unacknowledged for the knowledge, skills, and abilities they have accrued over a lifetime of experience.

Resilience is the development of mechanisms to help older people face the challenges associated with aging. It includes the presence of available resources and behaviors reflecting positive attitudes in the face of adversity in aging (Lima et al., 2023).

The physical and functional assessments of older adults should include inquiry about coping and adaptation in the face of stressors: What do you do when you face difficulties in life? How do you handle change in your life? What is your philosophy about life? Even more important to assess is the presence of mental, social, and physical resources to cope with adversity (MacLeod et al., 2016):

- Optimism, positive emotions, hopefulness

- Contact with family and friends, community involvement, sense of purpose, social support, positive relationships

- Independence, high mobility, physical health, self-rated successful aging

There is evidence to support the central role of religiosity and spirituality in well-being, health, and overcoming adversity. Inquiry about religious and spiritual values, beliefs, and practices are part of whole-person assessment and person-centered care (Buja et al., 2024; Coelho et al., 2022; Lima et al., 2020; MacKinlay, 2022; Oz et al., 2022; Shaw et al., 2016; Thauvoye et al., 2018).

Interprofessional Collaboration and Caregiving

Older adults benefit greatly from interprofessional teams working collaboratively on improving health outcomes (Cadet et al., 2024; Wei et al., 2022). Effective interprofessional teams embrace and utilize the following four competencies (Interprofessional Education Collaborative, 2023):

- Values and ethics: Work with team members to maintain a climate of shared values, ethical conduct, and mutual respect.

- Roles and responsibilities: Use the knowledge of one's own role and team members' expertise to address individual and population health outcomes.

- Communication: Communicate in a responsive, responsible, respectful, and compassionate manner with team members.

- Teams and teamwork: Apply values and principles of the science of teamwork to adapt one's own role in a variety of team settings.

Patient care quality is a major outcome of interprofessional collaboration. Measurable beneficial outcomes are patient satisfaction; patient and family education (medication adherence, medication reconciliation, nutrition counseling, self-management skills); reduced readmission rates, illness complications, and emergency wait times; and care transition and discharge follow-up.

Quality of Life in Aging

The World Health Organization (WHO) defines quality of life (QOL) as "an individual's perception of their position in life in the context of the culture and value systems in which they live and in relation to their goals, expectations, standards and concerns" (WHO, n.d.).

This all-encompassing definition of *quality of life* is mirrored in the United Nations' Sustainable Development Goal 3 (UNSDG 3), which is to "ensure healthy lives and promoting well-being for all at all ages" (UN, n.d.). Moreover, the human rights and worth of older adults is recognized in the United Nations (UN) adopted resolution, *UN Principles for Older Persons* (United Nations, 1991). Independence, participation, care, self-fulfillment, and dignity are core principles essential to programs, services, and government agencies providing care for older adults. Application and integration of these core principles within individual health professional practice and health care programs and services within communities demonstrate accountability in upholding the human rights of older adults (see Appendix A).

Quality of life in Aging:
Integration Across Practice, Communities, and Governments

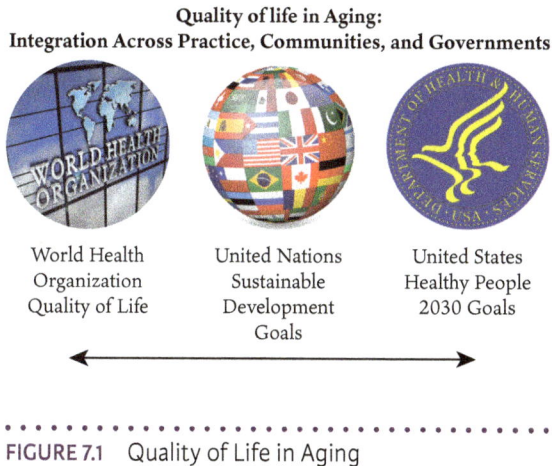

| World Health Organization Quality of Life | United Nations Sustainable Development Goals | United States Healthy People 2030 Goals |

FIGURE 7.1   Quality of Life in Aging

Aligned with UNSDG 3 are the Healthy People 2030 goals of the U.S. Department of Health and Human Services, Office of Disease Prevention and Health Promotion. Healthy People 2030 (HP 2030) identifies overarching goals for the health and well-being of older adults (USDHHS, n.d.-a). The Healthy People initiative began in 1980 with 10-year objectives for improving health and well-being nationwide. Measurable objectives, tools to track progress, and end of decade assessments are continually monitored and disseminated (USDHHS, n.d.-d). Health care practitioners can use this tool to search objectives, leading health indicators relevant to older adults, and progress toward goal achievement in their own communities. Additionally, several evidence-based tools and resources for assessment, evaluation, and planning care of older adults are readily available (see Appendix B).

The Social Determinants of Health (SDOH) are core aspects of the U.S. Healthy People 2030 objectives. The SDOH consist of five domains: (1) economic stability, (2) education access and quality, (3) health care access and quality, (4) neighborhood and built environment, and (5) social and community context (USDHHS, n.d.-b; USDHHs, n.d.-c).

The SDOH for older adults are specifically relevant in all five domains, considering the previous discussion of potential stressors:

- Older adults with lower incomes are more likely to have disabilities.

- Social isolation and loneliness are associated with a higher risk of dementia and other health problems; positive social relationships contribute to longer and healthier lives.

- Older adults may struggle with digital literacy in using and understanding medical documents, which affects ability to make well-informed health decisions.

- Older adults have chronic health conditions, which affects their access to affordable, quality health care. Lack of health care in rural areas, high out-of-pocket costs, and transitions from private insurance to Medicare often complicate older adults' care.

- Accessible neighborhoods and a built environment with convenient access to grocery stores and safe places to get active become increasingly important for older adults with decreased mobility.

Other aspects of quality of life are personal safety, creative expression, opportunity to help and encourage others, participation in public affairs, socialization, and leisure. Health-related quality of life focuses regarding people's level of ability, daily functioning, and ability to experience a fulfilling life (International Society for Quality of Life Research, n.d.) include:

- Disease

- Injury

- Impairment

- Health perceptions

- Health care and treatments

- Policy

Assessment of quality of life in older adults is helpful in targeting age- and population-specific interventions. An essential document in the literature is the World Health Organization Quality of Life Survey (WHOQOL-100; WHO, n.d.). The WHOQOL-100 has six major domains and facets: (1) physical capacity, (2) psychological, (3) level of independence, (4) social relationships, (5) environment, and (6) spirituality/religion/personal beliefs. An overall measure is that of overall quality of life and general health perceptions. An abbreviated form of the WHOQOL-100 is available. Both forms have been back translated into multiple languages by researchers employing the tools.

The Social Vulnerability Index (SVI) is another indicator of quality of life. Social vulnerability refers to the potential negative effects on communities caused by external stresses on human health, such as natural or human-caused disasters or disease outbreaks. Reducing social vulnerability can decrease both human suffering and economic loss. The Centers for Disease Control (CDC) and the Agency for Toxic Substances and Disease Registry (ATSDR) have created a place-based index and database that map, identify, and quantify persons experiencing social vulnerability.

The Minority Health SVI is an extension of the CDC/ATSDR SVI that includes additional community characteristics of social vulnerability, such as demographic variables, health care access, and chronic disease prevalence contributing to social vulnerability (https://minorityhealth.hhs.gov/minority-health-svi). The Minority Health SVI also identifies those communities that will need assistance before, during, and after a public health emergency.

Social vulnerability is determined by an index that is calculated from selected indicators (variables). The index is used to rank counties and determine the relative vulnerability of each community compared to other communities. The Minority Health SVI provides the relative vulnerability of each county.

The CDC/ATSDR SVI includes indicators specific to the Minority Health SVI:

- Socioeconomic status
- Household characteristics
- Racial and ethnic minority status
- Housing type and transportation
- Health care infrastructure and access
- Medical vulnerability

An equally important discussion relating to wellness and quality of life is that of caregiving at the end of life. Open discussions about the dying process and end of life care have become an increasingly important issue in health care.

End of Life Caregiving

Death is the cessation of all biological functions. Death may ultimately result from chronic illness and its complications, debilitating and terminal disease, severe trauma, complications of treatment interventions, or natural causes. Caregiving at the end of life is focused on helping the older adult maintain their dignity—ensuring their comfort, preferences (including cultural, traditional, and Indigenous practices), and needs (physical, emotional, social, and spiritual) are met. It is understanding and respecting their decisions about their own care. Clear explanations and open communication are important. Activity tolerance and energy conservation are also important considerations. At times the dying person may wish to engage in usual activities and patterns, including socialization with family, relatives, and friends. The dying process remains in the background of awareness. At other times the dying process will be at the forefront of active care as biological processes cease and the body begins to shut down. The older adult at end of life may experience a range of emotions and physical sensations. Withdrawal, restlessness, and disorientation are emotional experiences that caregivers have observed. Increased sleepiness, skin coolness, incontinence, decreased urine output, altered respiration, and decreased food and fluid intake are physical signs and symptoms of the dying process.

Palliative care seeks to alleviate symptoms of severe illness through comfort measures versus curative measures. Hospice focuses on care during the period closest to death; generally, persons with 6 months or less to live are placed on hospice care. Both palliative care and hospice care focus on symptom alleviation. Patients and their families benefit from education and access to both types of care. The health care team is responsible for providing or navigating access to resources and ensuring individuals and family members, who are often caregivers, receive needed support. In addition to nurses, physicians, pharmacists, and nutritionists, composition of the health care team is contingent upon patient need to maintain dignity and quality of life at end of life. Team composition may include occupational and physical therapists, mental health professionals, and social workers. Social workers have knowledge of community resources and can navigate patients and families through the complexities of health care insurance and coordinate care across delivery systems. Tangible support may take the form of pain medication, oxygen, and specialized equipment such as a hospital bed, wheelchair, walker or other mobility aids, and assistive health care personnel to help with activities of daily living such as bathing, showering, and meal preparation. Home health, palliative care, and hospice nurses provide continuous assessment and reassessment and interventions as the patient's needs change. Parenteral medication administration, care of complex wounds, and invasive venous access devices are some examples of direct care provided in home hospice care. Nurses advocate for patients and their families and work collaboratively with the health care team. Psychological and spiritual support may be provided through counseling with a mental health professional or someone the patient views as a spiritual guide, be it a priest, pastor, monk, Indigenous healer, a prayer group, or a support group.

The needs of family members, sometimes an older adult spouse, who often take on the roles and responsibilities of in-home hospice caregivers, must not be overlooked. Family caregivers often experience strain and overlook their own health and self-care needs. Providing respite care for the in-home caregiver prevents caregiver strain while the health care team attends to or arranges care for the older adult at end of life. Respite care can be arranged at a facility or within the home. The family caregiver can then take care of their own medical care appointments; take needed time to participate in recreational leisure activities; socialize with other family, relatives, and friends; or access needed mental health or spiritual care. Participation in virtual or in-person support groups facilitated by a qualified health care professional may be a helpful resource for the caregiver.

Introducing and raising a discussion about end of life planning and end of life care remains yet a sensitive topic for health care professionals, patients, and their families. Nonetheless, health care professionals have a responsibility to patients to discuss end of life issues. Nurses, in particular, as reflected in the American Nurses Association (ANA) Code of Ethics (see Chapter 1), "practices with compassion and respect for the inherent dignity, worth, and unique attributes of every person."

In many health care facilities, it is common to ask patients if they have an advance health care directive. Under the Patient Self Determination Act (PDSA) of 1990, patients with capacity have the right to give instructions about their health care and to name someone else to make health care decisions on their behalf. Advance directives are the patient's statements of their own wishes and directions to others before the need arises. Health care providers therefore must inform patients of their right to make decisions concerning their medical care, document this information in the medical record, not discriminate against persons who have an advance directive, and educate staff and community about advance directives.

A person designates another person to act on their behalf through a power of attorney (POA), a legal document. A general POA allows a named person to make financial decisions under specific circumstances. A durable POA allows a named person rights and responsibilities to make health care–related decisions when persons cannot do so for themselves.

Physician's Order for Life Sustaining Treatment (POLST) is a medical order completed by the health care provider and the patient based on open and rich dialogue about the patient's medical care, beliefs and values, and treatment goals. It is supplementary to an advance directive. The POLST involves both a communication process and a form. States have their own POLST programs and forms. For example, in California, the POLST treatment categories include cardiopulmonary resuscitation (CPR); medical interventions; artificially administered nutrition information; signatures, including the patient's signature or that of their legally recognized decision maker; and HIPAA disclosure to other health care providers as necessary. Patient completion of the POLST form is voluntary.

A valuable education and training resource is the End of Life Nursing Education Consortium (ELNEC). The consortium is a national and international collaborative educational initiative with the City of Hope in Duarte, California, and the American Association of Colleges of Nursing (AACN) to improve and advance palliative care. Resources on the consortium website include publications, simulations, patient teaching resources, and faculty tools (AACN, n.d.). Curricular integration of competencies ensures that graduates are prepared to provide effective and compassionate end of life care to diverse groups of patients.

The Conversation Project is another valuable resource to begin conversations about end of life wishes. The project is a public engagement initiative of the Institute for Healthcare Improvement (IHI). The initiative encourages everyone to talk about their care wishes through the end of life so that they are understood and respected. The project website contains tool kits, research publications, guidelines for community engagement, videos, and curricular, community, and faith-based resources for clinicians, caregivers, patients, and their family members.

Chapter Summary

This chapter has provided a brief overview about key concepts and normal age-related changes, wellness and illness prevention, quality of life, and end of life care. Evidence-based assessment tools and resources for end of life planning and care have been introduced to the reader. Also noted is the necessity for collaborative and interprofessional teamwork in maintaining wellness in aging and through the end of life.

Glossary

12-lead electrocardiogram (EKG or ECG): A noninvasive test to determine cardiac activity. Attachments (removable gel electrodes) are placed on the patient's anterior chest wall and upper and lower extremities. The attachments are connected to a machine that records electrical activity of the heart as waveforms. The recording helps diagnose regularities, irregularities in heart rate and rhythm, or cardiac muscle damage.

Acid-base balance: Acid-base balance is the body's regulatory mechanism to help maintain homeostasis. This is measured as pH, or the concentration of hydrogen ions in a solution, such as blood or body fluids. The pH value ranges from 0 to 14; a pH value of 7.0 is neutral. The pH indicates whether a solution (such as a blood sample, arterial or venous) is acidic (acidosis) or alkaline (alkalosis). Normal blood pH values range from 7.35–7.45. The two body systems that help regulate pH are the respiratory and renal systems. Oxygenation status can also be determined from arterial or venous blood samples.

Alveoli: Terminal end units of the respiratory tree. Anatomically, the trachea ("wind pipe") branches to form the right and left bronchi. These in turn branch into bronchioles, and finally alveoli. Alveoli are air sacs surrounded by a rich capillary network. Gas exchange of oxygen and carbon dioxide occurs at the alveolar level.

Alzheimer's disease: A neurodegenerative disease characterized by an increased number of beta amyloid proteins, or plaques surrounding the neurons, and an accumulation of tau proteins within the neurons, or neurofibrillary tangles. The neurons are progressively deprived of nutrients, and eventually cues of early, middle, or late stages of the disease are observable. Progressive damage to the brain occurs, particularly in that area where memories are stored.

Angina: Pain resulting from constriction or blockage of one or more of the coronary arteries that supply the cardiac muscle. Blockage results from atherosclerosis (plaque) within the coronary artery lining or an embolus (clot). The coronary arteries are responsible for supplying the heart with oxygen and nutrients. Branches are the left main, left anterior descending, the circumflex, and the right coronary arteries.

Autoregulation: The intrinsic ability of an organ to adapt and maintain its blood supply in response to demands or workload. For example, organs such as the brain, muscles, and kidney are able to regulate blood flow in proportion to the need for oxygen and other nutrients. Autoregulation is also affected by the autonomic nervous system, consisting of the sympathetic and parasympathetic systems. The sympathetic system responds to stressful or dangerous situations ("fight or flight" reaction), essentially putting the body on alert. The parasympathetic system function is opposite that of the sympathetic system and is responsible for internal functions when at rest.

B lymphocytes: B lymphocytes are part of the body's immune system. B lymphocytes are white blood cells that make proteins known as antibodies. When an antigen is detected (a threat or pathogen such as bacteria, virus, or parasite), B lymphocytes produce antibodies to destroy pathogens. The B lymphocyte develops from stem cells. The B lymphocyte system is fully developed at birth, and after birth they are developed in the bone marrow.

Blood pressure: The amount of force (arterial pressure) exerted by the blood against an area of the vessel wall. It is measured in millimeters of mercury (mm Hg). Cardiac output (volume of blood pumped by the heart in one minute) and total peripheral resistance (the amount of force exerted on circulating blood by the vasculature of the body) affect blood pressure. Peripheral vascular resistance is determined by length and diameter of blood vessels and blood viscosity. Blood pressure is measured noninvasively by auscultation or an electronic device. A blood pressure reading consists of two numbers: (a) the systolic blood pressure, the first number, which measures the pressure the blood is pushing against your artery walls when the heart beats, and (b) the diastolic blood pressure, the second number, which measures the pressure the blood is pushing against the artery walls while the heart muscle rests between beats.

Brain natriuretic peptide (BNP): BNP is a protein that is a type of hormone that controls the cells of certain organs. The heart releases BNP into the bloodstream. It is measured through a blood sample. Elevated BNP levels indicate the heart is working harder to pump blood throughout the body. Since BNP is excreted through the kidneys, an elevated BNP level may also be an indicator of renal problems.

Cardiac enzymes: Substances released into the bloodstream when the heart muscle (myocardium) is damaged or stressed. Cardiac enzymes or biomarkers help diagnose, assess risk of, and manage acute myocardial infarction (MI, or "heart attack"), a life-threatening condition. In an acute MI, the person experiences sudden onset of persistent chest pain radiating to one or both arms, shoulders, stomach, or jaw, along with shortness of breath, nausea, sweating, and dizziness. Troponin, aspartate aminotransferase (AST), lactate dehydrogenase (LDH), myoglobin, creatine kinase (CK), and specifically the cardiac isoenzyme CK-MB are released from damaged myocardium. Levels of enzymes are measured through a blood sample obtained by venipuncture. The appearance, peak levels, and their resolution or normalization varies with each type of enzyme. However, treatment should not be delayed.

Cardiac stress test (or exercise stress test): A test to determine how the heart performs under work. The patient is asked to walk a treadmill or ride a stationary bike, which makes the heart work progressively harder. During testing the patient is attached to other equipment that measures heart rate, respirations, and EKG. The patient is closely monitored by a health care professional. The test is helpful in identifying coronary artery disease.

Cerebrospinal fluid (CSF): Cerebrospinal fluid is a clear, colorless fluid that circulates around the brain and spinal cord; it acts as a cushion. Cerebrospinal fluid can be analyzed for the presence of different substances or to help diagnose the presence of infection, autoimmune disease, cerebral bleeding, Alzheimer's disease, or tumors. It is obtained through a special invasive procedure known as a lumbar puncture or spinal tap.

Chest X-ray: A non-invasive imaging test that uses X-ray to examine the structures and organs in the chest and how well the heart and lungs are functioning or responding to treatment. A chest X-ray is also known as a chest radiograph. Certain heart problems, diseases, and traumatic injuries can cause changes in the structure of the heart or lungs. The patient will be asked to remove clothing, jewelry, or other objects that may get in the way of the test, and will be given a gown to wear. The patient stands or sits in front of the X-ray plate. The patient will be asked to take a deep breath and hold it for several seconds. Holding the breath after inhaling helps the heart and lungs show up more clearly on the image. While the patient is holding their breath, the image is taken. Chest X-ray uses a very small dose of ionizing radiation to produce images of the heart and lungs and the rib cage, or skeletal structure. Ionizing radiation is a type of energy released by atoms in the form of electromagnetic waves or particles.

Chronic obstructive pulmonary disease (COPD): A lung disease resulting in restricted airflow and difficulty breathing. Persons may have bronchitis or emphysema or both. Bronchitis is chronic irritation or inflammation in the airways. Thick mucus develops in the airway linings and blocks the airway passages. Emphysema is the destruction or collapse of the alveolar cellular walls or air sacs. Cough, sometimes with mucus; difficulty breathing; wheezing; and fatigue are signs and symptoms. Multiple factors contribute to COPD: smoking; air pollution; exposure to secondhand smoke; occupational exposure to dusts, fumes, or chemicals; indoor air pollution (biomass fuel, wood, animal dung, crop residue, or coal is used for cooking and heating in low- and middle-income countries); high levels of smoke exposure; poor growth in utero, prematurity, and frequent or severe respiratory infections in childhood that prevent maximum lung growth; childhood asthma; and a rare genetic condition called alpha-1 antitrypsin deficiency responsible for COPD at a young age.

Complete blood count (CBC): A blood test used to help identify and diagnose numerous conditions, response to treatment, and monitoring of overall health status. A blood sample is obtained from the patient through a venipuncture. The sample is analyzed for a battery of blood components: hemoglobin, hematocrit, red blood cell count (RBC), white blood cell count (WBC), platelets, and cell morphology. Hemoglobin carries oxygen, white cells constitute the immune system, and platelets are necessary for coagulation and hemostasis. Normal values are age-determined.

Continuous positive airway pressure (CPAP): A continuous positive airway pressure (CPAP) machine is a medical device that delivers a constant gentle flow of pressurized air into the nose or mouth to keep airways open during sleep. Continuous positive airway pressure therapy is prescribed to treat sleep-related breathing disorders like obstructive sleep apnea, in which tissues in the mouth and throat narrow or close your airways, causing breathing to stop for more than 10 seconds, then restarts. This breathing cycle occurs multiple times while sleeping. Daytime fatigue, concentration and memory problems, and morning headache result from airway obstruction during sleep. A CPAP machine includes a mask to fit over the nose or mouth, or both, tubing to connect the mask to the machine's

motor, and a motor that blows positive pressure (air) into the tube.

Dementia: A neurocognitive impairment characterized by progressive loss of memory, disorientation, impaired communication, concentration, and judgment. Behavioral and personality changes in advanced stages result in mood swings, aggressiveness, wandering, and confusion, all of which result in an inability to carry out activities of daily living. Causes of dementia are multifactorial and include neurodegenerative, vascular, and autoimmune disorders; traumatic brain injuries; and strokes.

Diabetes: A disorder in which carbohydrates, fats, and proteins are not metabolized for energy or fuel. The islet cells in the pancreas produce a hormone, insulin, which is necessary to move glucose into the cells for metabolism. In type 1 diabetes, an autoimmune disorder, the pancreas is unable to produce insulin as a result of the destruction of pancreatic beta cells. In type 2 diabetes, there is a peripheral tissue resistance to the effects of insulin resulting in hyperinsulinemia and hyperglycemia. Type 2 diabetes occurs in middle-aged to older adults.

Ejection fraction: An index of function of the left ventricle of the heart. It is the proportion of blood ejected during contraction compared with total ventricular filling (or the total amount of blood in the ventricle before contraction). A normal value is approximately 65% (or 0.65) of the total volume in the ventricle ejected with each contraction.

Fundoscopic exam: A noninvasive visualization of the interior of the eye using an instrument called an ophthalmoscope. Namely the retina, the innermost lining of the eye, is examined. The retina contains photoreceptors, rods, and cones that receive visual stimuli, which are in turn transmitted to the optic nerve. A funduscopic exam enables the visualization of the arteries, veins, optic nerve, and other abnormalities indicative of health problems such as hypertension, diabetes, and glaucoma.

Gas exchange: the physiological process of airflow or ventilation into and out of the alveoli and perfusion of blood flow to alveolar capillaries; ventilation and perfusion allow for the exchange of oxygen and carbon dioxide

Glomerular filtration rate (GFR): A gauge to assess the filtering function of the kidneys. The nephron, the functioning unit that filters waste, is surrounded by a capillary network called the glomerulus. The glomerulus is enclosed in a sac, Bowman's capsule. As blood filters through the glomerulus (glomerular filtrate or the ultrafiltrate), unwanted substances are filtered and excreted in the urine; wanted substances are reabsorbed back into the bloodstream. The glomerular filtration rate is the quantity of filtrate formed each minute in all nephrons of the kidneys. Normal values are approximately 125 milliliters per minute.

Heart failure: A state in which the heart functions inefficiently as a pump; blood flowing from the ventricles to the systemic circulation is insufficient to meet oxygenation and metabolic needs. Heart failure can involve either the right or left ventricle or both and can result in enlargement of the heart and volume overload. Volume overload is the increased retrograde hydrostatic pressure from the ventricles into the pulmonary or peripheral circulation. In right-sided heart failure, for example, systemic venous congestion is seen in the extremities (edema or swelling of the extremities). In left-sided heart failure, dyspnea (shortness of breath), coughing, and pulmonary edema (pulmonary congestion) are present.

Hypertension (high blood pressure): Hypertension occurs when the force flowing through blood vessels is consistently high. Blood pressure is defined as the pressure or force of blood pushing against blood vessel walls. As the heart contracts and ejects its volume, it encounters peripheral resistance of the vessel walls of the circulatory system. Blood pressure is measured in millimeters of mercury (mm HG) and consists of two numbers: the systolic pressure (or the top number), which measures when the heart contracts, and the diastolic pressure (or the bottom number), when the heart is relaxing between beats. The American College of Cardiology and the American Heart Association recommend a goal of less than 130/90 for those at least 65 years of age (Vemu et al., 2024). Hypertension, uncontrolled and untreated, affects all organ systems.

Hyperthyroidism: A condition in which there is an excess of circulating thyroid hormones in the body due to an autoimmune disorder or pituitary or thyroid gland tumors. All body systems are affected by this hypermetabolic state. Manifestations include heat intolerance, irritability, restlessness, goiter (enlarged thyroid gland), tachycardia (heart rate greater than 100), palpitations, increased blood pressure, weight loss, increased appetite, diarrhea, visual changes, and menstrual irregularities.

Hypothalamic-pituitary-adrenal (HPA) axis: A feedback system of neurohormones (chemical messengers) produced by the hypothalamus and the pituitary and adrenal glands. The HPA axis is responsible for maintaining homeostasis (a stable state) and managing the body's response to stressors. The hypothalamus is located at the base of the brain, and below it is the pituitary gland. The adrenal glands are located above the kidneys. The hypothalamus responds to internal (physical, physiological, psychological) and external (environmental) signals. The hypothalamus secretes corticotropin-releasing hormone (CRH) and arginine vasopressin (AVP). These hormones are then transported to the anterior pituitary gland, which in turn secretes adrenocorticotropic hormone (ACTH). Adrenocorticotropic hormone stimulates the cortex of the adrenal glands to secrete yet another hormone, cortisol. Cortisol increases blood glucose and manages protein, fat, and carbohydrate metabolism. When adequate levels of cortisol are detected in the bloodstream, the brain signals the hypothalamus to stop the release of CRH and AVP; it also signals the pituitary gland to produce less ACTH.

Hypothyroidism: A condition caused by a deficiency in thyroid

hormone. Thyroid hormone production is regulated by a feedback system involving the hypothalamus, the anterior pituitary gland, and the thyroid gland. The thyroid gland is located in front of the neck. Thyoptropin-releasing hormone in the hypothalamus stimulates the anterior pituitary to secrete thyroid-stimulating hormone (TSH); subsequently, TSH stimulates the thyroid cells to release thyroid hormones, known as T3 and T4. Triiodothyronine, or T3, is the active form of thyroid hormone. Tetraiodothyronine, or T4, when released into the circulation, converts to T3. Manifestations of hypothyroidism include fatigue, lethargy, decreased short-term memory, palpitations, intolerance to cold, gait disturbances, weight gain, and constipation. These manifestations in older adults may go undiagnosed and untreated, leading to more serious, life-threatening conditions.

Intraocular pressure: A measurement of the fluid pressure contained within the eye. The fluid contained within the eye (aqueous and vitreous humor, or bodily fluid) is necessary for vision and nourishment. Intraocular pressure is measured in several ways, the most common being a noninvasive procedure called air puff tonometry. The person is seated and positioned on a chin rest in front of a machine that directs a puff of air to flatten the cornea. The greater the force needed to flatten the cornea the higher the intraocular pressure. Normal intraocular pressure ranges from 10 to 20 mm Hg. Increased intraocular pressure can lead to a condition known as glaucoma, in which there is damage of the optic nerve and the retinal artery and loss of vision.

Meninges: Three layers of membrane that envelop the brain and spinal cord. The layers are the pia mater, arachnoid mater, and dura mater. The pia mater follows every surface of the brain and spinal cord. The arachnoid mater is a gauzelike sleeve of connective tissue outside the pia mater. The dura mater is a collagenous membrane external to the arachnoid, and a subdural space lies between these two membranes. The meninges are supported by a vascular network. Cerebrospinal fluid circulates around the meninges, brain, and spinal cord; it provides cerebral protection, nourishment, and waste removal.

Myocardial infarction (MI): A myocardial infarction is also referred to as a "heart attack." The coronary arteries are the main blood supply to the heart. With occlusion, or coronary artery disease, the myocardium is deprived of oxygen. Myocardial cell damage and tissue damage occur. These changes are detected through an EKG and the presence of cardiac enzymes.

Peristalsis: The involuntary contraction and relaxation of longitudinal and circular muscles throughout the digestive tract, which allows for the propulsion of contents in the gastrointestinal tract.

Pressure ulcer: Breakdown of skin resulting in injury. Pressure ulcers are also referred to as "decubitus ulcers," "pressure sores," or "bedsores." The skin and soft tissue injuries occur as a result of prolonged pressure and shear over bony prominences. They vary in characteristics and severity. The extent and depth of injury is classified by stages. While the etiology of pressure ulcers is multifactorial, they are *preventable*. Person-centered care includes identification and assessment of risk factors, implementation of appropriate interventions and treatments, continuous monitoring and evaluation, and patient, family, and staff education.

Serum electrolytes: Minerals present in body fluids that have important functions in maintaining acid-base balance, muscle and nerve function, and heart rate and rhythm. Electrolytes supply cellular nutrients, remove cellular waste, and are important to bone health. The electrolytes, which are normally obtained from food and fluids, are sodium, potassium, bicarbonate, chloride, calcium, magnesium, and phosphate. Electrolyte levels are measured through a blood test.

Serum lipids: Lipids are fatty chemical compounds that are essential to body functions. These are phospholipids, triglycerides, and cholesterol. They are found in cell membranes and hormones. Lipids store energy, control cellular activity and transport, and aid in vitamin absorption. Lipids are measured through a blood test and include total cholesterol, low-density lipoprotein (LDL) and high-density lipoprotein (HDL) cholesterol, and triglycerides. A high total cholesterol and LDL levels (sometimes referred to as "bad" cholesterol), along with high triglyceride levels, are associated with an increased risk of cardiovascular disease. High levels of HDL (sometimes referred to as "good" cholesterol) is associated with a lower risk of cardiovascular disease. A level of 60 mg/dL (milligrams per deciliter) or higher is considered desirable. Person-centered care includes interpretation of diagnostic lab tests; health goals and actions for prevention and reducing risk; and consideration of treatment interventions.

Stroke (cerebrovascular accident [CVA]): Loss of brain function resulting from blockage of vessels (from a clot or fatty deposits) that supply oxygen and nutrients to the brain; a hemorrhage, or a break in the blood vessels (from trauma or injury) also reduces oxygen and nutrient delivery to the brain. The neurological, cognitive, and psychomotor deficits associated with a stroke correspond to the part of the brain that was traumatized, injured, or deprived of oxygen.

Synapse: The junction between neurons (nerve cells). Neurotransmitters ("chemical messengers"), produced in a cell body, diffuse across the synapse and bind with specific receptors on a target cell that generates an action or change in the target cell (ex: a muscle contraction, release of a hormone). The brain has approximately 86 billion neurons that communicate with each other through electrochemical signals. Neurotransmitters control many important bodily functions:

- Acetylcholine (ACh)
- Norepinephrine (NE)
- Dopamine (DA)
- Serotonin (5-HT)

- Other common neurotransmitters include other catecholamines, gamma-aminobutyric acid (GABA), glycine, and glutamic acid.

T lymphocytes: A type of white blood cell that provides immunity by destroying pathogens. The most common T lymphocytes are the CD4+ T cells (helper T cells) and CD8+ T Cells (cytotoxic T cells, or killer T cells). T lymphocytes recognize and bind to protein receptor antigens of infected cells or cancer cells and destroy them. Activated helper T-cells signal other immune cells to rid the body of invading cells.

Traumatic brain injury (TBI): An injury occurring to the brain as a result of a forceful blow or jolt to the head or a penetrating object, explosion, or assault. Falls in older adults can result in TBI. Persons experience physical, cognitive, and perceptual changes. Physical changes include headache, seizures, vision and hearing changes, pupillary inequalities, cerebrospinal fluid drainage from the nose or ears, nausea, vomiting, slurred speech, weakness, loss of balance, and fatigue. Cognitive changes include loss or change in consciousness, confusion, difficulty remembering or concentrating, mood swings, and difficulty sleeping. Manifestations of TBI may be short- or long-term. Complications of TBI are cerebral hemorrhage, cerebral edema (swelling), and skull fracture. It is important to seek immediate medical attention and follow-up.

Villi: Fringe-like mucus-producing projections that line the mucosal wall of the small intestine. They absorb water, electrolytes, carbohydrates, fats, and proteins.

Visual acuity: The sharpness or clarity of vision at a distance. It is evaluated by having a patient read letters on a chart at a distance of 20 feet. Persons with normal vision, or "20/20," can see the same amount of detail 20 feet away as the average person. In hyperopia, or farsightedness, persons can see at a distance but not close objects. In myopia or nearsightedness, persons can see close up but not at a distance.

Appendix A: United Nations Principles for Older Persons

Adopted by General Assembly resolution 46/91 of 16 December 1991
The General Assembly,

Appreciating the contribution that older persons make to their societies,

Recognizing that, in the Charter of the United Nations, the peoples of the United Nations declare, inter alia, their determination to reaffirm faith in fundamental human rights, in the dignity and worth of the human person, in the equal rights of men and women and of nations large and small and to promote social progress and better standards of life in larger freedom,

Noting the elaboration of those rights in the Universal Declaration of Human Rights, the International Covenant on Economic, Social and Cultural Rights and the International Covenant on Civil and Political Rights and other declarations to ensure the application of universal standards to particular groups,

In pursuance of the International Plan of Action on Ageing, adopted by the World Assembly on Ageing and endorsed by the General Assembly in its resolution 37/51 of 3 December 1982,

Appreciating the tremendous diversity in the situation of older persons, not only between countries but within countries and between individuals, which requires a variety of policy responses,

Aware that in all countries, individuals are reaching an advanced age in greater numbers and in better health than ever before,

Aware of the scientific research disproving many stereotypes about inevitable and irreversible declines with age,

Convinced that in a world characterized by an increasing number and proportion of older persons, opportunities must be provided for willing and capable older persons to participate in and contribute to the ongoing activities of society,

Mindful that the strains on family life in both developed and developing countries require support for those providing care to frail older persons,

Bearing in mind the standards already set by the International Plan of Action on Ageing and the conventions, recommendations and resolutions of the International Labour Organization, the World Health Organization and other United Nations entities,

Encourages Governments to incorporate the following principles into their national programmes whenever possible:

Independence

1. Older persons should have access to adequate food, water, shelter, clothing and health care through the provision of income, family and community support and self-help.

2. Older persons should have the opportunity to work or to have access to other income-generating opportunities.

3. Older persons should be able to participate in determining when and at what pace withdrawal from the labour force takes place.

4. Older persons should have access to appropriate educational and training programmes.

5. Older persons should be able to live in environments that are safe and adaptable to personal preferences and changing capacities.

6. Older persons should be able to reside at home for as long as possible.

Participation

7. Older persons should remain integrated in society, participate actively in the formulation and implementation of policies that directly affect their well-being and share their knowledge and skills with younger generations.

8. Older persons should be able to seek and develop opportunities for service to the community and to serve as volunteers in positions appropriate to their interests and capabilities.

9. Older persons should be able to form movements or associations of older persons.

Care

10. Older persons should benefit from family and community care and protection in accordance with each society's system of cultural values.

11. Older persons should have access to health care to help them to maintain or regain the optimum level of physical, mental and emotional well-being and to prevent or delay the onset of illness.

12. Older persons should have access to social and legal services to enhance their autonomy, protection and care.

13. Older persons should be able to utilize appropriate levels of institutional care providing protection, rehabilitation and social and mental stimulation in a humane and secure environment.

14. Older persons should be able to enjoy human rights and fundamental freedoms when residing in any shelter, care or treatment facility, including full respect for their dignity, beliefs, needs and privacy and for the right to make decisions about their care and the quality of their lives.

Self-fulfilment

15. Older persons should be able to pursue opportunities for the full development of their potential.

16. Older persons should have access to the educational, cultural, spiritual and recreational resources of society.

Dignity

17. Older persons should be able to live in dignity and security and be free of exploitation and physical or mental abuse.

18. Older persons should be treated fairly regardless of age, gender, racial or ethnic background, disability or other status, and be valued independently of their economic contribution.

🌀 Appendix B: Evidence-Based Tools for Assessment and Care of Older Adults

GeriatricPain.org

https://geriatricpain.org/pacslac-ii

Chan, S. Hadjistavropoulos, T., Wiliams, J., Lints-Martindales, A., (2014). Evidence-based development and initial validation of the Pain Assessment Checklist for Seniors with Limited Ability to Communicate-II (PACSLAC-II) [Instructions]. *The Clinical Journal of Pain, 30*(9), 816–824. https://geriatricpain.org/sites/geriatricpain.org/files/2020-06/PACSLAC%20II%20Checklist%20Instructions.pdf

Chan, S. Hadjistavropoulos, T., Wiliams, J., Lints-Martindales, A., (2014). Pain Assessment Checklist for Seniors with Limited Ability to Communicate-II (PACSLAC-II) *The Clinical Journal of Pain, 30*(9), 816–824 https://geriatricpain.org/sites/geriatricpain.org/files/2020-06/PACSLAC%20II%20Checklist.pdf

Glasgow Coma Scale: https://www.glasgowcomascale.org/

Hartford Institute for Geriatric Nursing. (n.d.). *Try this series.* https://hign.org/consultgeri-resources/try-this-series

United States Department of Health and Human Services (USDHHS). (n.d.). *Evidence-based resources related to older adults.* Healthy People 2030. https://health.gov/healthypeople/objectives-and-data/browse-objectives/older-adults/evidence-based-resources

Montreal Cognitive Assessment (MoCA). https://mocacognition.com/

MOCA Cognition. (n.d.). *Montreal cognitive assessment.* https://geriatrictoolkit.missouri.edu/cog/MoCA-8.3-English-Test-2018-04.pdf

MOCA Cognition. (n.d.). *Pain assessment in advanced dementia scale (PAINAD).* https://geriatrictoolkit.missouri.edu/cog/painad.pdf

International Parkinson and Movement Disorder Society (MDS). (n.d.). *Clinical outcome assessments.* https://www.movementdisorders.org/MDS/MDS-Clinical-Outcome-Assessment.htm#assessments

Consult respective copyright holders for permissions to reproduce tools and the literature for administration and interpretation of results. Older adults should contact their primary health care provider or other qualified health care professional for further information, guidance, interpretation of assessment results, and care.

Appendix C: ACT III: Your Plan for Aging in Place

National Aging in Place Council (NAIPC)

Welcome. This template is designed to help you make your own plan for Aging in Place.

Aging in Place is a rapidly growing lifestyle option for Americans approaching or beyond retirement age. It facilitates remaining in the home of your choice for as long as you would like as opposed to relocating to a nursing home or other medical facility. You are able to do this because the services you need to live a secure and safe life are now available to you in your home.

In order to successfully age in place we strongly recommend some planning. And this template will make planning easy for you.

This will take a chunk of time. We estimate about an hour. But you don't have to do it all in one sitting. You can save your responses, take a break, and come back. You might want to involve your family or trusted advisors in this process. Make it fun, make it an occasion. Invite them to join you around the dining room table and answer the questions together.

Using This Template

We are going to walk you through the essential concerns to sustain a safe and secure lifestyle in your home. We are going to ask a lot of questions you need to ask yourself. The questions are primarily about what you now have and what you might need.

The key areas we are going to evaluate are:

- Housing
- Health and wellness
- Personal finance
- Transportation
- Community and social interaction
- Education and entertainment

At the end of each section, you will find space entitled "My Needs." Here, you fill in your needs in that area.

"My Needs" Evaluation

When you complete answering the questions in all of the areas, you will be given a "My Needs Summary." This summary will provide you with resources and information on the areas that you may need assistance, based on your answers to the questions. When you complete this template, you should have a clearer picture of your own future.

After receiving your "My Needs Summary," we will provide you with a "My Needs Evaluation." If you have a local Chapter in your community, a member of the Chapter will assess your "My Needs Summary" to assist you with finding the resources and providers that you will need to age in place. If no local Chapter exists in your community, the NAIPC National staff will assist you with your "My Needs Evaluation."

If an event occurs in your future that alters your circumstances (a change in location, a financial gain or loss, a health issue, etc.), we recommend you revisit your plan to determine if you need to do some rethinking.

So now let's begin to go through the essentials of your lifestyle and evaluate your circumstances.

Housing

Choice of Residence

Are you comfortable in your current residence?   Yes   No

Would you like to remain in your current residence for as long as possible?
                                                          Yes   No

What is it that most makes you want to remain in your current residence?
____Location   ____Familiarity   ____Size   ____Accessibility to family
____Accessibility to friends

Comfort & Accessibility

Can you comfortably move around your home?   Yes   No

If not, have you considered or researched home modifications?   Yes   No

Personal Home Assessment

Please check one of the following:

❏ **My current home is comfortable, safe and affordable for me**

❏ **My current home is not comfortable enough, safe enough, affordable enough**

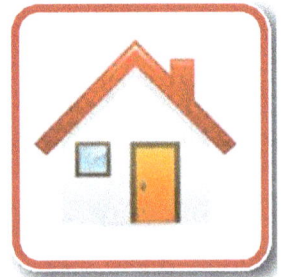

If your current home is not comfortable, safe or affordable, what changes are you considering?_____

_____

My Housing Needs: _____

Health and Wellness

General

On a scale of 1–10, where 10 is "Excellent" and 1 is "Poor," how would you rate your overall health?

     1   2   3   4   5   6   7   8   9   10

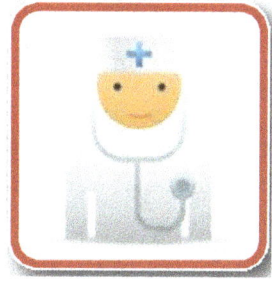

What concerns do you have in particular about your health?

- ❑ Medical Condition/Chronic Illness
- ❑ Chronic Pain
- ❑ Limited mobility
- ❑ Costs of medical care
- ❑ Difficulty getting to doctor's appointments

Daily Living/In Home Care

Are you able to independently perform daily activities? Check all that you are still able to perform:

- ❑ Bathing and showering
- ❑ Personal hygiene and grooming *(including washing hair)*
- ❑ Dressing
- ❑ Eating/feeding
- ❑ Functional mobility *(moving from one place to another while performing activities)*
- ❑ Personal device care
- ❑ Toilet hygiene *(completing the act of relieving oneself)*

Do you have a family member or friend who can serve as your caregiver and assist you with these activities?   Yes   No

Do you have the financial resources to hire a caregiver to assist you with your daily activities?   Yes   No

Health and Wellness

If you were to experience a major health problem (surgery, diagnosis with chronic illness, etc.), do you have a plan for how you will pay for your medical expenses?   Yes   No

Have you completed the appropriate legal medical documents, including a healthcare power of attorney, a living will, and an advanced directive?   Yes   No

If not, do you have information on how to complete these documents?   Yes   No

My Health & Wellness Needs: _____

Personal Finance

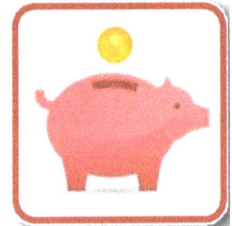

Do you currently have sufficient income and or/savings to cover your monthly expenses?   Yes   No

Are you concerned you will not have enough money to cover your expenses for the remainder of your life?

         Yes   No

Have you prepared a list of your income and assets and your expenses?   Yes   No

Do you get advice on how to utilize your savings or pension?   Yes   No

Whom do you depend on for advice?

- ❑ Professional financial advisor
- ❑ Family
- ❑ Friends
- ❑ Banker

My Personal Finance Needs: _____

Transportation

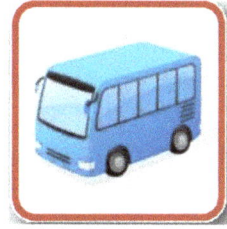

Do you have a plan in place for your future transportation needs if your ability to drive changes?   Yes   No

Have you set aside money for your potential future transportation needs?   Yes   No

My Transportation Needs:_____

Community & Social Interaction

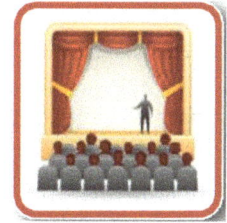

Do you feel that you have enough social interaction with other people?   Yes   No
If you answered "no", what are the reasons? *(Select all that apply)*

- ❏ Transportation

- ❏ Home is isolated

- ❏ Children/family no longer live in the area

Do you feel that you are a part of your local community?   Yes   No

My Community & Social Interaction Needs:_____

My Needs Summary
My Housing Needs:

_____

_____

_____

My Health & Wellness Needs:

_____

_____

_____

My Personal Finance Needs:

_____

_____

_____

My Transportation Needs:

_____

_____

_____

My Community & Social Interaction Needs:

_____

_____

_____

My Priority List

Things I can accomplish myself:

1. _____
2. _____
3. _____
4. _____
5. _____
6. _____
7. _____
8. _____

9. _____

10. _____

Things for which I need help and support:

1. _____

2. _____

3. _____

4. _____

5. _____

6. _____

References

American Association of Colleges of Nursing (AACN). (n.d.). *End of life nursing education consortium (ELNEC).* https://www.aacnnursing.org/elnec

American Geriatrics Society Beers Criteria Update Panel. (2023). American Geriatrics Society 2023 updated AGS Beers Criteria for potentially inappropriate medication use in older adults. *Journal of the American Geriatrics Society, 71*(7), 2052–2081. https://doi.org/10.1111/jgs.18372

Boss, G. R., & Seegmiller, J. E. (1981). Age-related physiological changes and their clinical significance. *The Western Journal of Medicine, 135*(6), 434–440.

Buja, A., Grotto, G. & Vo, D. (2024). Association of religiosity and spirituality with survival among older adults: A systematic review. *Journal of Public Health.* https://doi.org/10.1007/s10389-024-02303-1

Cadet, T., Cusimano, J., McKearney, S., Honaker, J., O'Neal, C., Taheri, R., Uhley, V., Zhang, Y., Dreker, M. & Cohn, J. S. (2024). Describing the evidence linking interprofessional education interventions to improving the delivery of safe and effective patient care: A scoping review. *Journal of Interprofessional Care, 38*(3), 476–485. https://doi.org/10.1080/13561820.2023.2283119

Centers for Disease Control and Prevention (CDC). (n.d.). *Recommended vaccines for adults.* https://www.cdc.gov/vaccines-adults/recommended-vaccines/index.html

Coelho-Júnior, H. J., Calvani, R., Panza, F., Allegri, R. F., Picca, A., Marzetti, E., Alves, V. P. (2022). Religiosity/spirituality and mental health in older adults: A systematic review and meta-analysis of observational studies. *Frontiers in Medicine, 9.* https://doi.org/10.3389/fmed.2022.877213

Hartford Institute for Geriatric Nursing (HIGN). (n.d.). *Try this series: Best practices of care for older adults.* NYU Rory Meyers College of Nursing. https://hign.org/consultgeri-resources/try-this-series

Interprofessional Education Collaborative (IPEC). (2023). *IPEC core competencies for interprofessional collaborative practice: Version 3.* https://www.ipecollaborative.org/2021-2023-core-competencies-revision

International Society for Quality of Life Research (ISOQOL). (n.d.). *What is quality of life?* Retrieved July 2, 2024, from https://www.isoqol.org/what-is-qol/

Lima, G. S., Figueira, A. L. G., de Carvalho, E. C., Kusumota, L., & Caldiera, S. (2023). Resilience in older people: A concept analysis. *Healthcare, 11*, 2491. https://doi.org/10.3390/healthcare 11182491

Lima, S., Teixeira, L., Esteves, R., Ribeiro, F., Pereira, F., Teixeira, A., & Magalhães, C. (2020). Spirituality and quality of life in older adults: A path analysis model. *BMC Geriatrics, 20*, 1–8.

MacKinlay, E. (2022). A narrative of spirituality and ageing: Reflections on the ageing journey and the spiritual dimension. *Religions, 13*(5), 463. https://doi.org/10.3390/rel13050463

MacLeod, S., Musich, S., Hawkins, K., Alsgaard, K., & Wicker, E. R. (2016). The impact of resilience among older adults. *Geriatric Nursing, 37*(4), 266–272. https://doi.org/10.1016/j. gerinurse.2016.02.014

National Institute of Neurological Disorders and Stroke. (n.d.). *NIH Stroke scale.* National Institutes of Health. https://www.ninds.nih.gov/health-information/stroke/assess-and-treat/ nih-stroke-scale

Shaw, R., Gullifer, J., & Wood, K. (2016). Religion and spirituality: A qualitative study of older adults. *Ageing International, 41*, 311–330.

Thauvoye, E., Vanhooren, S., Vandenhoeck, A., & Dezutter, J. (2018). Spirituality and well-being in old age: Exploring the dimensions of spirituality in relation to late-life functioning. *Journal of Religion and Health 57*, 2167–2181. https://doi.org/10.1007/s10943-017-0515-9

United Nations (n.d.) *United Nations: The 17 goals.* https://sdgs.un.org/goals

United Nations. (1991). *United Nations principles for older persons.* https://www.ohchr.org/en/ instruments-mechanisms/instruments/united-nations-principles-older-persons

United States Department of Health and Human Services (USDHHS). (n.d.-a). *Healthy people 2030: Older adults.* Office of Health Promotion and Disease Prevention. https://health.gov/ healthypeople/objectives-and-data/browse-objectives/older-adults

United States Department of Health and Human Services (USDHHS). (n.d.-b). *Healthy people 2030: Social determinants of health.* Office of Health Promotion and Disease Prevention. https:// health.gov/healthypeople/priority-areas/social-determinants-health

United States Department of Health and Human Services (USDHHS). (n.d.-c). *Healthy people 2030: Social determinants of health and older adults.* Office of Health Promotion and Disease Prevention. https://health.gov/our-work/national-health-initiatives/healthy-aging/ social-determinants-health-and-older-adults

United States Department of Health and Human Services (USDHHS). (n.d.-d). *History of healthy people.* https://odphp.health.gov/our-work/national-health-initiatives/healthy-people/ about-healthy-people/history-healthy-people

Vemu, P. L., Yang, E., & Ebinger, J. (2024). *2023 ESH hypertension guideline update: Bringing us closer together across the pond.* American College of Cardiology. https://www.acc.org/ Latest-in-Cardiology/Articles/2024/02/05/11/43/2023-ESH-Hypertension-Guideline- Update

Wei, H., Horns, P., Sears, S. F., Huang, K., Smith, C. M., & Wei, T. L. (2022). A systematic meta-review of systematic reviews about interprofessional collaboration: facilitators, barriers, and outcomes. *Journal of Interprofessional Care, 36*(5), 735–749. https://doi.org/10.1080/135618 20.2021.1973975

World Health Organization (WHO). (n.d.). *WHOQOL: Measuring quality of life.* https://www. who.int/tools/whoqol

Selected Bibliography

Abayomi, S. N., Sritharan, P., Yan, E., Saripella, A., Alhamdah, Y., Englesakis, M., Tartaglia, M. D., He, D., & Chung, F. (2024). The diagnostic accuracy of the Mini-Cog screening tool for the detection of cognitive impairment—A systematic review and meta-analysis. *PLoSOne, 19*(3), 1–16.

Administration for Community Living. (2022). *2021 profile of older Americans.* U.S. Department of Health and Human Services, Administration on Aging. https://acl.gov/sites/default/files/Profile%20of%20OA/2021%20Profile%20of%20OA/2021ProfileOlderAmericans_508.pdf

Administration for Community Living. (2024). *Aging in the United States: A strategic framework for a national plan on aging.* ICC Report to Congress. https://acl.gov/sites/default/files/ICC-Aging/StrategicFramework-NationalPlanOnAging-2024.pdf

Agency for Health Care Research and Quality (AHRQ). (2023). *National healthcare quality and disparities report.* https://www.ahrq.gov/research/findings/nhqrdr/nhqdr23/index.html

Alberts, B., Johnson, A., Lewis, J., Raff, J., Roberts, K., & Walker, P. 2002). Lymphocytes and the cellular basis of adaptive immunity. In B. Alberts (Ed.), *Molecular biology of the cell* (4th ed.). 1-1616. Garland Science: New York. Available from: https://www.ncbi.nlm.nih.gov/books/NBK26921/

Allen, M. J., & Sharma, S. (2023, August 8). Physiology, adrenocorticotropic hormone (ACTH). In *StatPearls.* StatPearls Publishing: Florida. 1-7. https://www.ncbi.nlm.nih.gov/books/NBK500031/

Ammaturo, D. A., Hadjistavropoulos, T., & Williams, J. (2017). Pain in dementia: Use of observational pain assessment tools by people who are not health professionals. *Pain Medicine, 18*(10), 1895–1907. https://doi.org/10.1093/pm/pnw265

Arevalo-Rodriguez, I., Smailagic, N., Roqué-Figuls, M., Ciapponi, A., Sanchez-Perez, E., Giannakou, A., Pedraza, O. L., Bonfill Cosp, X., & Cullum, S. (2021). Mini-mental state examination (MMSE) for the early detection of dementia in people with mild cognitive impairment (MCI). *Cochrane Database of Systematic Reviews.* https://doi.org/10.1002/14651858.CD010783.pub3

Brady, D., Kohler, U., & Zheng, H. (2023). Novel estimates of mortality associated with poverty in the US. *JAMA Intern Med, 183*(6), 618–619. https://jamanetwork.com/journals/jamainternalmedicine/article-abstract/2804032

Can Oz, Y., Duran, S., & Dogan, K. (2022). The meaning and role of spirituality for older adults: A qualitative study. *Journal of Religion & Health, 61*(2), 1490–1504. https://doi.org/10.1007/s10943-021-01258-x

Centers for Disease Control (n.d.). *Health literacy: Older adults.* https://www.cdc.gov/healthliteracy/developmaterials/audiences/olderadults/index.html

Chan, S., Hadjistavropoulos, T., Williams, J., & Lints-Martindale, A. (2014). Evidence-based development and initial validation of the pain assessment checklist for seniors with limited ability to communicate-II (PACSLAC-II). *The Clinical Journal of Pain, 30*(9), 816–824. https://doi.org/10.1097/AJP.0000000000000039

Chu, B., Marwaha, K., Sanvictores, T., Ayoola, O.A., & Ayers D. (2024), May 7). Physiology, stress reation. In *StatPearls.* StatPearls Publishing, Treasure Island, Florida, 1-11. https://www.ncbi.nlm.nih.gov/books/NBK541120/

Davis, K. L., & Davis, D.D. (2023, July 17). Home safety techniques. In *StatPearls.* StatPearls Publishing. Treasure Island, Florida. 1-4. https://www.ncbi.nlm.nih.gov/books/NBK560539/

Dunlavey C. J. (2018). Introduction to the hypothalamic-pituitary-adrenal axis: Healthy and dysregulated stress responses, developmental stress and neurodegeneration. *Journal of Undergraduate Neuroscience Education, 16*(2), R59–R60. https://www.ncbi.nlm.nih.gov/pmc/articles/PMC6057754/

Flanagan, B. E., Hallisey, E. J., Adams, E., & Lavery, A. (2018). Measuring community vulnerability to natural and anthropogenic hazards: The Centers for Disease Control and Prevention's Social Vulnerability Index. *Journal of Environmental Health, 80*(10), 34–36.

Frances Payne Bolton School of Nursing. (n.d.). Quality and Safety Education for Nurses (QSEN), 2012. Graduate QSEN competencies. Case Western University. https://www.qsen.org/competencies-graduate-ksas

Garbarino, S., Lanteri, P., Bragazzi, N. L., Magnavita, N., & Scoditti, E. (2021). Role of sleep deprivation in immune-related disease risk and outcomes. *Communications Biology, 4*(1), 1304. https://doi.org/10.1038/s42003-021-02825-4

Hartford Institute for Geriatric Nursing. (n.d.) *Curriculum map with AACN competencies.* https://hign.org/consultgeri-resources/guides-and-competencies/competencies

Hassani, P., Izadi-Avanji, F. S., Rakhshan, M., & Majd, H. A. (2017). A phenomenological study on resilience of the elderly suffering from chronic disease: A qualitative study. *Psychology Research and Behavior Management, 10*, 59–67. https://doi.org/10.2147/PRBM.S121336

Huffman, J. L., & Harmer, B. (2023, February 20). End-of-life care. In *StatPearls*. StatPearls Publishing: Treasure Island, Florida. 1-13. https://www.ncbi.nlm.nih.gov/books/NBK544276/

Hui, D., Nooruddin, Z., Didwaniya, N., Dev, R., De La Cruz, M., Kim, S. H., Kwon, J. H., Hutchins, R., Liem, C., & Bruera, E. (2014). Concepts and definitions for "actively dying," "end of life," "terminally ill," "terminal care," and "transition of care": A systematic review. *Journal of Pain and Symptom Management, 47*(1), 77–89. https://doi.org/10.1016/j.jpainsymman.2013.02.021

Integrative Therapeutics. (2017, April 11). *Hans Selye's general adaption syndrome and the HPA axis: Exploring the connection.* [Video]. YouTube. https://youtu.be/9FdmxfXrygA?si=eNEZVoCk-m2QoOWrM (play to 3:35 minutes)

International Society for Quality of Life Research (ISOQOL). (n.d.). *Who we are.* https://www.isoqol.org/who-we-are/

Interprofessional Education Collaborative. (n.d.). https://www.ipecollaborative.org/

Januszewski, J., Forma, A., Zembala, J., Flieger, M., Tyczyńska, M., Dring, J. C., Dudek, I., Świątek, K., & Baj, J. (2023). Nutritional supplements for skin health—A review of what should be chosen and why. *Medicina, 60*(1). https://doi.org/10.3390/medicina60010068.

Khaku, A. S., & Tadi, P. (2023, August 7). Cerebrovascular disease. In *StatPearls*. StatPearls Publishig: Treasure Island, Florida. 1-13. https://www.ncbi.nlm.nih.gov/books/NBK430927/

Khalili, H., Lackie, K., Langlois, S., da Silva Souza, C. M., & Wetzlmair, L. C. (2023). The status of interprofessional education (IPE) at regional and global levels—update from 2022 global IPE situational analysis. *Journal of Interprofessional Care, 38*(2), 388–393. https://doi.org/10.1080/13561820.2023.2287023

Kubler-Ross, E. (1969). *On death and dying: What the dying have to teach doctors, nurses, clergy, and their own families.* MacMillan.

Kutner, M., Greenberg, E., Jin, Y., & Paulsen, C. (2006). *The health literacy of America's adults: Results from the 2003 National Assessment of Adult Literacy.* National Center for Education Statistics. https://nces.ed.gov/pubsearch/pubsinfo.asp?pubid=2006483

Lima, G. S., Figueira, A. L. G., Carvalho, E. C., Kusumota, L., & Caldeira, S. (2023). Resilience in older people: A concept analysis. *Healthcare (Basel, Switzerland), 11*(18), 2491. https://doi.org/10.3390/healthcare11182491

Michalak, M., Pierzak, M., Kręcisz, B., & Suliga, E. (2021). Bioactive compounds for skin health: A review. *Nutrients, 13*(1), 203. https://doi.org/10.3390/nu13010203

Milman, L. H., Faroqi-Shan, Y., Corcoran, C. D., & Damele, D. M. (2018). Interpreting Mini-Mental State Examination performance in highly proficient bilingual Spanish-English and Asian Indian-English Speakers: Demographic adjustments, item analyses, and supplemental measures. *Journal of Speech, Language, and Hearing Research61*(4) 847–856.

Mode, N. A., Evans, M. K., & Zonderman, A. B. (2016). Race, neighborhood economic status, income inequality and mortality. *PLoS ONE, 11*(5), e0154535. https://doi.org/10.1371/journal.pone.0154535

National Academies of Sciences. (2020). *Social isolation and loneliness in older adults: Opportunities for the health care system.* The National Academies Press. https://doi.org/10.17226/25663

National Aging in Place Council (NAIPC). (n.d.). *Act III: Your plan for aging in place.* https://athomeaging.info/wp-content/uploads/2018/01/ACTIII-pdf2.pdf

National Heart, Lung, and Blood Institute. (n.d.). Sleep science and sleep disorders. https://www.nhlbi.nih.gov/science/sleep-science-and-sleep-disorders

National Institute on Aging. (n.d.). *Caregiving.* National Institutes of Health. https://www.nia.nih.gov/health/caregiving

National Institute on Aging. (n.d.). *Elder abuse.* National Institutes of Health. https://www.nia.nih.gov/health/elder-abuse

National Institute on Aging. (n.d.). *Loneliness and social isolation—Tips for staying connected.* National Institutes of Health. https://www.nia.nih.gov/health/loneliness-and-social-isolation/loneliness-and-social-isolation-tips-staying-connected

National Institute on Aging. (n.d.). *Stroke: Signs, causes, treatment.* National Institutes of Health. https://www.nia.nih.gov/health/stroke/stroke-signs-causes-and-treatment#what

National Institute on Aging. (n.d.). *Vaccinations and older adults.* https://www.nia.nih.gov/health/immunizations-and-vaccines/vaccinations-and-older-adults

National Institutes of Health Office of Dietary Supplements. (n.d.). *Vitamin B12, fact sheet for consumers.* https://ods.od.nih.gov/factsheets/vitaminb12-healthprofessional/

National POLST Coalition. (n.d.). *POLST for health care professionals.* https://polst.org/professionals-page/

Patient Self Determination Act of 1990, H.R.5067—101st Congress. (1990, November 5). https://www.congress.gov/bill/101st-congress/house-bill/5067

Parkinson's Foundation. (n.d.). *What is Parkinson's?* https://www.parkinson.org/understanding-parkinsons/what-is-parkinsons

Riva, M. M. (2024). *Home safety for older adults: A comprehensive guide 2024.* National Council on Aging. https://www.ncoa.org/adviser/sleep/home-safety-older-adults/

Roth, T. (2007). Insomnia: definition, prevalence, etiology, and consequences. *Journal of Clinical Sleep Medicine, 3*(5 Suppl), S7–S10.

Schagen, S. K., Zampeli, V. A., Makrantonaki, E., & Zouboulis, C. C. (2012). Discovering the link between nutrition and skin aging. *Dermato-endocrinology, 4*(3), 298–307. https://doi.org/10.4161/derm.22876

Seadler, B. D., Toro, F., & Sharma, S. (2023). *Physiology, alveolar tension physiology, alveolar tension.* National Library of Medicine, National Center for Biotechnology Information. https://www.ncbi.nlm.nih.gov/books/NBK539825/

Selye, H. (1950, June 17). Stress and the general adaptation syndrome. *British Medical Journal, 1*(4667), 1384–1392

Shah, S. J., Hoffman, A., Pierce, L. & Covinsky, K. E. (2023). Development and applicability of a risk assessment tool for hospital-acquired mobility impairment in ambulatory older adults. *Journal of the American Geriatrics Society.* https://doi.org/10.1111/jgs.18456

Taylor, J. A., Greenhaff, P. L., Bartlett, D. B., Jackson, T. A., Duggal, N. A., & Lord, J. M. (2023). Multisystem physiological perspective of human frailty and its modulation by physical activity. *Physiological Reviews, 103*(2), 1137–1191. https://doi.org/10.1152/physrev.00037.2021

Teoli, D., & Ghassemzadeh, S. (2023, Aug 28). Patient self-determination act. In *StatPearls*. StatPearls Publishing: Treasure Island, Florida. 1-5. https://www.ncbi.nlm.nih.gov/books/NBK538297/

U.S. Department of Health and Human Services (USDHHS). (n.d.). Evidence based resources for older adults. *Healthy People 2030*. https://health.gov/healthypeople/objectives-and-data/browse-objectives/older-adults/evidence-based-resources

Wei, H., Corbett, R. W., Ray, J., & Wei, T. L. (2019). A culture of caring: the essence of healthcare interprofessional collaboration. *Journal of Interprofessional Care, 34*(3), 324–331. https://doi.org/10.1080/13561820.2019.1641476

Weinick, R. M., Carney, M. T., Milnes, T., & Bierman, A. S. (2023). *Optimizing health and function as we age: Roundtable report.* Agency for Healthcare Research and Quality (AHRQ). https://www.ahrq.gov/sites/default/files/wysiwyg/ncepcr/tools/healthy-aging-roundtable.pdf

Zorek, J. A., Ragucci, K. R., Eickhoff, J., Najjar, G., Ballard, J. F., Blue, A. V., Bronstein, L. R., Dow, A., Gunaldo, T. P., Hageman, H., Karpa, K. D., Michalec, B., Nickol, D., Odiaga, J., Ohtake, P. J., Pfeifle, A., Southerland, J. H., Vlasses, F. R., Young, V., & Zomorodi, M. (2022). Development and validation of the IPEC Institutional Assessment Instrument. *Journal of Interprofessional Education and Practice, 29*, 100553. https://doi.org/10.1016/j.xjep.2022.100553

Websites

CONNECTING AND CARING THROUGH VISIBILITY, INCLUSION, AND ADVOCACY

Adding Life to Years

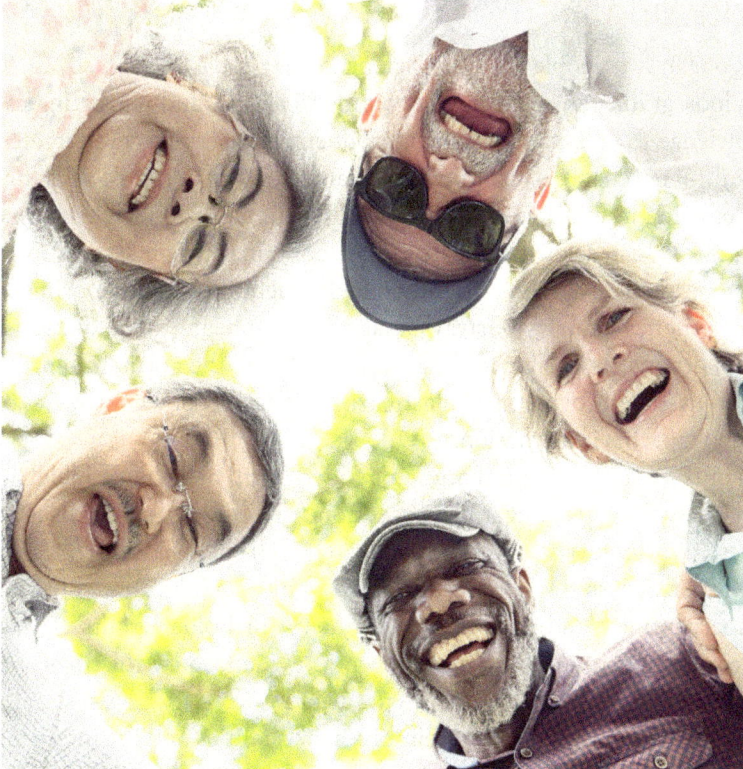

Image 8.1

Overview

This chapter explores ways to connect and care for older adults by heightening their visibility and inclusion, engaging their social participation, and utilizing their knowledge, skills, and abilities acquired over a lifetime.

Outcomes

The learner:

1. Understands the social context that contributes to ageism

2. Recognizes the need for older adults to actively utilize their abilities and to seek out new knowledge, skills, and experiences

3. Leverages the strengths, expertise, and insights of older adults in fostering and supporting their active engagement in their respective communities

4. Through reflective action, identifies and implements a change that supports the rights of older adults

Introduction

Globally, one in two people are ageist against older people (WHO, 2021b). One only needs to look at images, mass media communications, and marketing campaigns to acknowledge that consumer goods, products, and services are targeted toward more youthful populations. Clothing, for example, is not designed with the physical changes of aging in mind, but rather for the fashionable models who sport them. Greeting cards, such as birthday cards, often contain satiric messages toward older adults and perpetuate ageism rather than truly celebrating and honoring advancing age. The cosmetics industry portrays images of what beauty should look like. It has an array of products available to the consumer to defy the normal changes of aging. Medical tourism for cosmetic or plastic surgery has become a growing choice for those who want this intervention.

Ageism is socially accepted and embedded in all aspects of society. When it is taught at a young age, negative perceptions of aging reinforce discrimination, prejudices, and stereotypes. Ageism can also be self-incriminating when messages communicated across the lifespan inform how older adults should think, be, and act. Misperceptions lead to negative actions toward older adults. The COVID-19 pandemic is a prime example of ageism as evidenced by the disproportionate adverse impact on older adults. Ageism permeates societal systems—legal, medical, educational, and political. Ageism reinforces inequalities and the intergenerational divide, and limits opportunities to fully participate in society and enjoy basic human rights and personal freedoms.

A report of an independent expert submitted to the United Nations Human Rights Council (UNHRC; Mahler, 2021; UNHRC, 2021) clearly analyzes the pervasiveness of ageism and recommends interventions for prevention, promotion, and protection of the rights of older persons. Ageism perpetuates other inequalities (ableism, racism, sexism, and discrimination against LGBTQ+ persons). The media and its use of idioms about older adults further embed negative attitudes and continue to reinforce "isms" across society.

Ageism is manifested in health care and long-term care (denial of medications, treatments, medical interventions, isolation, and ageist behavior and attitudes of health care providers). The absence of curricula in health professions education attests to the perceived unimportance of teaching this information. Ageism drives abuse and violence toward older adults in health care settings, homes, and public spaces, including the internet. Abusers are family members, caregivers, legal guardians, financial representatives, and government workers. Societal norms, mandatory retirement ages, stereotypes about work abilities, and age limits in recruitment prohibit the right of older adults to work.

Older adults are often excluded from social activities based on deeply rooted and pervasive stereotypes, which leads to further isolation. Once persons have left the paid labor workforce, they are at risk for poverty. Consequently, older adults are denied financial tools and services because of poverty and age limits.

Global digitalization has become mainstream and often the only way to access many social activities and services, including health care. Older persons may live in communities where there is limited access to technology, or for various reasons may not be able to afford it. This further contributes to a technological divide and exclusion of older adults.

A Global Spark of Change: Counteracting Ageism and Ageist Attitudes

A global movement has ignited and continues to spark change. As younger generations eventually grow into their older adult years, the work of previous generations who have come before them will change the negative societal myths and stereotypes of aging.

As noted in the previous chapter, in 1991 the United Nations declared a resolution, Principles for Older Persons, which was adopted by member states. Since this first declaration, there has been increasing focus on the needs of older adults, with 2021–2030 declared as the Decade of Healthy Aging (United Nations, n.d.). Four critical action areas are:

- Combatting ageism: changing how we think, feel, and act toward age and ageism

- Creating age-friendly environments: developing communities in ways that foster the abilities of older people

- Providing integrated care: delivering person-centered integrated care and primary health services responsive to older people

- Ensuring access to long-term care: providing older people who need it with access to quality long-term care

Visibility of Older Adults Through Data Disaggregation

Central to the critical action areas is the visibility of older adults in all aspects of society. Clearly, data collection about older adults must be disaggregated to identify issues and hear their voices; understand their situations, needs, and perspectives; and utilize and implement their recommendations across social systems to improve quality of life in older years.

There is a critical demand for disaggregated data about older adults in each of the Sustainable Development Goals (SDGs). Nonetheless, existing disaggregated data for priority indicators of older adults in each of the goals are helpful in driving change. There are 46 priority SDG indicators to make older adults visible (WHO, 2024). Five-year age group intervals separated by gender and other characteristics help monitor differences across age groups, monitor the extent to which goals are met by country, and inform evidence-based decisions. For example, governments and societies use disaggregated data in the following ways:

- Assess responsiveness and effectiveness of social protection systems.

- Implement strategies and programs to address chronic diseases, suicide, and homicide.

- Analyze household incomes below the median and expenditures on health.

- Determine participation rate of youth and adults in formal and nonformal education and training.

- Inform government reporting and policy decisions to improve services and support for those experiencing violence.

- Identify digital connectivity, as evidenced by those who own a cell phone and who use the internet.

- Identify the proportion of persons living in slums, informal settlements, or inadequate housing.

- Identify the proportion of people who feel safe walking alone where they live.

- Analyze the proportion of people satisfied with the experience of public services.

- Determine the proportion of people who believe decision-making is inclusive and responsive by age, by gender, and by persons with disabilities.

- Assess participation in the labor market through unemployment rates by gender, by age, and by persons with disabilities.

In the U.S., analogous to the SDGs are Social Determinants of Health (SDOH) and Healthy People 2030 (HP 2030) goals. Overarching goals of HP 2030 are to improve the health and well-being of all persons (United States Department of Health and Human Services [USDHHS], n.d.-a):

- Attain healthy, thriving lives and well-being free of preventable disease, disability, injury, and premature death.

- Eliminate health disparities, achieve health equity, and attain health literacy to improve the health and well-being of all.

- Create social, physical, and economic environments that promote attaining the full potential for health and well-being for all.

- Promote healthy development, healthy behaviors, and well-being across all life stages.

- Engage leadership, key constituents, and the public across multiple sectors to take action and design policies that improve the health and well-being of all.

The HP 2030 leading health indicators are measurable objectives specific to older adults and focus on reducing health problems and improving quality of life. Leading health indicators are general health, cognitive health (the dementias), foodborne illnesses, infectious disease, injury prevention, osteoporosis, respiratory disease, and sensory or communication disorders. To date, only baseline data is available for most of these indicators (general health, cognitive health, osteoporosis, respiratory disease, and sensory or communication disorders). Other leading health indicators have "developmental" status, which means they are a high priority with evidence-based interventions but reliable baseline data is not yet available.

Information about older adults from the leading health indicator database is useful in targeting interventions, programs, and policies. For example, the proportion of fall-related deaths among older adults increased from 64.4 deaths per 100,000 population aged 65 years or older in 2018 to 76.9 deaths per 100,000 population aged 65 years or older in 2022. This indicator is worsening based on the established target of 63.4 deaths per 100,000. These deaths resulted from *unintentional* falls and could have been prevented (USDHHS, n.d.-c).

Indicators in which established targets have been met, are improving, or exceeded are in preventive screening, accessing care, and management of chronic illness. In contrast, much work remains ahead to address those indicators in which there is little or no improvement, or that are worsening. These objectives are wait times for care, breast cancer screening, diabetic screening and education, health care provider communication, health care decision-making, mental health care, physical activity, housing, poverty, lifestyle choice, and health maintenance (USDHHS, n.d.-b). Data are disaggregated by age, race and ethnicity, gender orientation, disability, and other characteristics (presence of other chronic illness, education, marital status, veteran status, health insurance, income, and geography).

The coordination and collaboration between agencies and nation-states to measure health indicators is a massive and necessary undertaking. Nonetheless, knowing and understanding specific information about older adults can generate individual actions and steps toward improving quality of life in older years.

Visibility of Older Adults Through Interventions

Changing the narrative of ageism and its embeddedness in institutions requires intentional, persistent, and concerted work of all parties at many levels—individuals, groups, organizations, public and private sectors, societies, and governments.

PUBLIC SPACES AND SERVICES

Public spaces must ensure the safety, comfort, and accessibility needs of older adults. Well-lighted spaces, nonskid floors and surfaces, high visibility markings that denote a change in height such as uneven steps, handrails, and entrances and exits that push open and close easily while allowing for ease of access with mobility aids promote safe surroundings. High-visibility signage with graphics in readable font, especially around potentially hazardous materials, warn people who may be unaware of dangers. Ergonomic, sturdy, and comfortable furniture of appropriate height with armrests does much to support posture and balance. Elimination of barriers in high-traffic areas, such as furniture and area rugs that may prevent access or create the potential for falls, promote safety. Windows that allow for infusion of natural light and green plants add to both aesthetics and a sense of well-being.

Equipment used by older adults must meet safety and accessibility requirements. The U.S. Department of Justice, Civil Rights Division (https://www.ada.gov/), and the U.S. Department of Labor, Occupational Safety and Health Administration (https://www.osha.gov/) provide standards, guidance, and educational materials.

WORK FLEXIBILITY AND ADAPTATION

Older adults have the right to work and have access to the labor market (UNHRC, 2021), Many older adults in the U.S. continue to work well beyond the traditional retirement age, which may vary from 62 to 67 years. The literature has identified several critical determinants to continue working (Fiske & Becker, 2022):

- Health
- Education
- Financial literacy
- Employer-sponsored pensions
- Social security
- Wealth and income
- Rising debt
- Health insurance
- Family household structure
- Caregiving responsibilities
- Disability

In 2023, there were 11.2 million Americans age 65 or older in the labor force, either working or actively seeking work. In addition, 23.2% of men and 16% of women who were in the workforce were 65 years of age or older This is an increase of older adults in the workforce as compared to 2000 data, where 17.70% were men, and 9.40% were women who were 65 years of age or older (ACL, 2024). The Pew Research Center reports that older workers 65 years or older typically earned $22.00 in 2022, as compared to $13.00 in 1987. Approximately 9.0% of older adults in the workforce are 75 years of age or older, are more diverse, have higher education levels, and are healthier (Fry & Braga, 2023).

The presence of older adults in the workforce is not without its challenges. While older workers may be more cautious, occupational injuries are more fatal for those over 60 years of age (CDC, 2024a, 2024b). As noted in a previous chapter, many older adults have chronic conditions—most common are arthritis and hypertension—and may be present at work in spite of feeling ill. It is imperative that employers allow time for healing, adapt work conditions, and have preventive programs in place. Flexible work arrangements are particularly important, as older workers may also be caregivers for family members or significant others.

There are many positive benefits for retaining older adults in the workforce. Among these are their institutional knowledge, expertise, and strategic thinking. They may be better equipped to work well with coworkers and maintain low levels of stress on the job due to their experience and life skills. Opportunities for promotion or advancement, training and professional development, and recruitment processes should be age neutral (AHRC, 2021).

INTERGENERATIONAL CONTACT

Intergenerational contact fosters interaction between different generations and helps reduce ageism, including ageism against younger people. Intergenerational contact can happen through face-to-face interaction, gardening, art, or music. Interviews, discussions, and service learning or collaborative projects in school-based programs are a means of shaping positive encounters (WHO, 2021a). Workplace intergenerational teams are an opportunity for raising awareness of diverse perspectives, solving complex issues, and generating innovative and creative solutions. The quality and frequency of interactions are considerations in planning contact.

Educational interventions are effective instructional tools that provide knowledge, skills, and competencies in reducing ageism. These interventions can occur through reading, guest lectures, simulations, virtual reality, online learning, role-playing, reflection and journaling, community-based participatory action, and clinical rotations in health care settings (WHO, 2021a). Challenging stereotypes and prejudices by actively engaging learners may also foster empathy and compassion toward older adults. Clearly, an exploration of the learner's relationship with generations in their own families could also be a starting point for change and understanding.

MENTORING

Mentoring describes a formal or informal meaningful relationship in which an individual guides another's personal and professional growth; provides social, economic, and upward mobility opportunity; and influences the mentee's career trajectory toward goal achievement or success. The mentoring relationship involves effective communication and support for the mentee. The mentoring process can occur in any setting and may be long- or short-term.

Mentors are experienced role models; provide wisdom, counsel and caring support; serve as sponsor and navigator in organizations and institutions; and facilitate growth and development through appropriate challenges. Mentors are also aware of their limitations, responsibilities, and boundaries. Most of all, mentors enjoy the opportunity to pass on wisdom, knowledge, and collaboration with mentees (APA, 2024).

Older adults are positioned to mentor others effectively, as they have work experience, knowledge and expertise, life skills, and networks that have been cultivated over an extended period of time. It is helpful for mentor and mentee to have transparency, a clear sense of the relationship in terms of mutually established goals, realistic and feasible expectations, and time commitment. It may also be helpful to initially determine if mentor and mentee are a good match, and perhaps at some point determine if more than one mentor is helpful. Another mentor may have added skills sets that could enrich the mentee's growth and development.

LIFELONG LEARNING

Lifelong learning is a mindset. It is the continuous pursuit of knowledge, skills, and experiences that improve, enhance, or enrich one's own abilities, and to achieve or realize potential. Lifelong learning can be an intrinsic motivator, and therefore, any programs or outreach efforts must consider what older adults value. Lifelong learning can be formal or informal. Lifelong learning occurs in a variety of settings. Universities and community colleges offer adult completion programs that lead to a degree or certificate. Universities also have dedicated institutes that provide educational opportunities through lectureships or events. Other community organizations can provide a venue for lifelong learning through the performing arts (music, theater, dance) and literary art. Museums also provide a source of enrichment through visual art, education, and curated displays. Community colleges are in a position offer to workshops and resources in acquiring practical skills. Parks and recreation departments and community programs that cater to older adults are other venues for lifelong learning activities.

Inclusion of *all* older adults in stimulating and engaging learning benefits individuals, families, and community well-being, regardless of socioeconomic status, ethnicity, education, or work. Among the benefits of lifelong learning are personal and professional growth, continuance of meaningful and purposeful work, self-confidence, self-sufficiency, improvement in cognitive function, mental health, and social connectedness.

Visibility of Older Adults Through Research Inclusion

The scientific literature is replete with information about aging and older adults, with an emphasis on disease. While there is ongoing research about many variables affecting disease and curative interventions, underrepresented and ethnic minority groups have been largely excluded from research participation. Research findings cannot be generalized to underrepresented and ethnic minority groups. Optimum care for diverse older adults includes best evidence, quality, and transparency. Person-centered, older adult care is not achievable when American Indian/Alaska Natives, Asian Pacific Islanders, Latinos, and African Americans are excluded from research.

As persons age differently, distinct age categories in studies may detect differences and changes. For example, findings in persons who are 60–65 years of age may be different from findings aggregated for persons 60–70 years of age. There may be also differences among "superagers," older adults who have above average memory skills for their age. Studies that report results for discrete categories of superagers, (80–85 years, 86–91 years, and 92–97 years, vs. 80–90 years) may yield helpful information.

Research has also addressed mental health in older adults, mainly on depression and social isolation. There is also research about post-traumatic stress in older immigrant populations. Absent in current studies is inquiry into those social, cultural, spiritual, and contextual factors that have contributed to their survivorship, sustenance, resilience, and generativity, or continued willingness to help ensure the well-being of younger generations.

The barriers and facilitators of conducting research with older adult populations require further exploration. While research studies are approved through appropriate academic and health care institutions, the conduct of research and its outcomes may not always be for the greater good of the intended participants. This may lead to distrust and hesitancy to participate in future research studies, or even refusal. There are many considerations throughout the research process in working with older adults, including underrepresented and ethnic minority older age groups and communities of color:

STUDY PURPOSE

- What is the study's purpose and its relevance to individuals, groups, and the community?

- Is the purpose communicated clearly in easily understandable language to potential study participants of diverse and underrepresented groups?

- Does the study and its variables have meaning to individuals, groups, and the community?

RECRUITMENT

- What forethought is given to the recruitment and participation of older adults and their health status, mobility, energy, and endurance levels?

- What will study participants be asked to do that may compromise their health, such as invasive procedures, or endurance, such as responding to a battery of tests?

- What logistical considerations will be in place, such as transportation; scheduling; convenience, including pre- and post-testing events; or repeated measures or assessments over time intervals?

INFORMED CONSENT

- Who has the capacity to give informed consent to participate in the research study?

- Are there permissions to be sought from community leaders such as a spiritual or tribal leader, a council of elders, or a respected community liaison?

- Are there cultural, spiritual, or Indigenous rituals that by tradition should occur prior to implementation of the study?

- What assessments and considerations have been made concerning potential study participants' information literacy, health literacy, and digital literacy?

- Are the benefits and risks of study participation clearly explained in language that is easily understood?

- What assurances are there that communication and data collection tools (such as consent forms, surveys, tests) that have been translated are valid and culturally and linguistically appropriate?

INCENTIVES

- Have considerations about fair and reasonable incentives for participation been carefully weighed given the study logistics?

DATA COLLECTION

- What accommodations will be made during data collection should there be gender-sensitive issues, questions, physical examinations, or invasive test procedures?

RESEARCH DISSEMINATION

- How are study participants informed of research results?

- Are results to research participants clearly communicated and explained in an understandable manner?

- How are study participants involved in communicating research findings to others in their community?

- Are study participants involved in the evaluation of study successes and limitations?

- How are study participants involved in the sustainability of positive benefits or positive study outcomes?

POST-RESEARCH AND SUSTAINABILITY

- Upon completion of the study, how are positive study benefits or outcomes made accessible and available to individuals, groups, and the community?

- If interventions have proved to be effective and successful, are the interventions also made available to control groups, or those who did not receive an intervention?

- Are there benefits in providing education or skills?
- Are there ethical considerations of withholding an intervention post-research from those who could directly benefit from it?

Visibility of Older Adults Through Advocacy

Advocacy is a vehicle to change the negative narrative of ageism. This can be accomplished at the personal, interpersonal, community, or organizational levels. Self-awareness at the personal level is a firm beginning step. Attending to one's own word choices or speech in verbal, written, and electronic communications conveys respect and disarms negativity. Misperceptions, inappropriate references, and colloquialisms about older adults in interpersonal interactions can be met with starting a conversation about what people understand and believe, and subsequently deeper conversations may ensue, leading to the acquisition of valid facts and knowledge resources (WHO, 2021a).

Many organizations have mission and vision statements that declare their values. Organizations desire that values are visible and manifested among employees or their representatives in providing services. Organizations can decrease ageism by attending to employee awareness about ageism. This can be accomplished through educational workshops, campaigns, internal and external communications, and policies and practices that inform how employees interact with older adults and how older persons readily access quality of life–enhancing activities and services (UNITAR, 2023, 2024; Phoenix, 2020). Nonprofit global networked organizations have valuable contributions in helping communities advance the rights of older adults through education and training programs (Cavatore et al., 2021).

Chapter Summary

In summary, this chapter has identified ways in which to make older adults visible in society. Data disaggregation, intergenerational contact, lifelong learning, research inclusion, and advocacy are specific ways to heighten visibility of older adults, whether alone or in combination. A concerted and sustained effort is needed for meaningful change.

Glossary

Ageism: The adherence to stereotypes, prejudice, and discrimination on the basis of age, which is directed toward others or self, and is manifested in behaviors, practices, or processes.

Ageist: One who maintains stereotypic views, prejudice, and discrimination against an age group, especially elderly persons.

Data disaggregation: Separation of data to examine its component parts to identify individual or unique characteristics, attributes, behaviors, or outcomes.

Global digitalization: Conversion by countries of information into digital form, which impacts daily living at many levels, such as health care access and services, education, labor and employment, communication, transportation, economy, finance, and social programs. The extent to which global digitalization is in place varies by high-, middle-, and low-income countries and by their ability to implement technology infrastructure and to adapt to evolving and rapidly emerging technologies.

Incentive: A token given arbitrarily by researchers to research participants for participation in studies. This may take many forms, such as a gift card, a chance at a drawing, transportation support, or some other services rendered in-kind.

Informed consent: Critical communication and exchange of information between the researcher or investigator and potential research participants prior to initiation of a research study. Informed consent, founded upon ethical principles of respect for autonomy and nonmaleficence, consists of the following required elements for the protection of human participants: The participant is competent and capable of giving consent; is an autonomous agent; has the opportunity to choose what will/will not happen to them; is given full disclosure and details in understandable language about the research procedure or what they will be asked to do; has the right to refuse participation or withdraw from the study at any time without any retaliation; has the opportunity to ask questions; is given information about how their confidentiality, privacy, and data will be protected. The potential participant then makes an informed decision to participate/not participate in the study. The informed consent process is documented, and a record of the above information is provided to the participant who has voluntarily agreed.

Intergenerational contact: Shared interaction and communication among persons of varying generations, such as that between younger and older persons. This may take the form of working together on a project, mentoring or helping one another to learn new skills or tasks, or sharing knowledge and experiences in an atmosphere of respect. There is no emphasis on differences in position or roles that make one or the other more authoritative or vulnerable.

Intergenerational divide: Opinions, beliefs, and values held among persons of varying generations, such as that between younger and older persons. Adherence to these thoughts and ideas can lead to misunderstanding, miscommunication, divisiveness, isolation, stereotypes, prejudice, and discrimination.

Lifelong learning: An ongoing, continued, and evolving pursuit of knowledge, skills, abilities, and experiences throughout one's life. Such a pursuit may be through formal or informal learning to refine, develop, or hone in on foundations that already exist, or to seek out experiences and challenges that are altogether new or different.

Social protection systems: Systems, policies, and programs designed by governments that are intended as safety nets to provide assistance and protection across the life cycle of individuals and families, and for its vulnerable citizens during crises and shocks. These systems, aligned with human rights, vary by country and population needs. Examples of social protection systems and programs in the U.S. are Medicare, Medicaid, Social Security, unemployment, employment injury, family and child support, maternity, and disability benefits.

Superagers: Persons over 80 years of age who have cognitive performance better than individuals who are decades younger. Characteristics of superagers include less age-related cognitive decline and structural brain changes; they remain physically and mentally active seek out stimulation and challenges, and have satisfying, high-quality relationships.

Appendix A: A Reminiscence Interview Exemplar

Reminiscing with Dee*

Contributed by Christina Felice M. Yap, BSN, RN PCCN

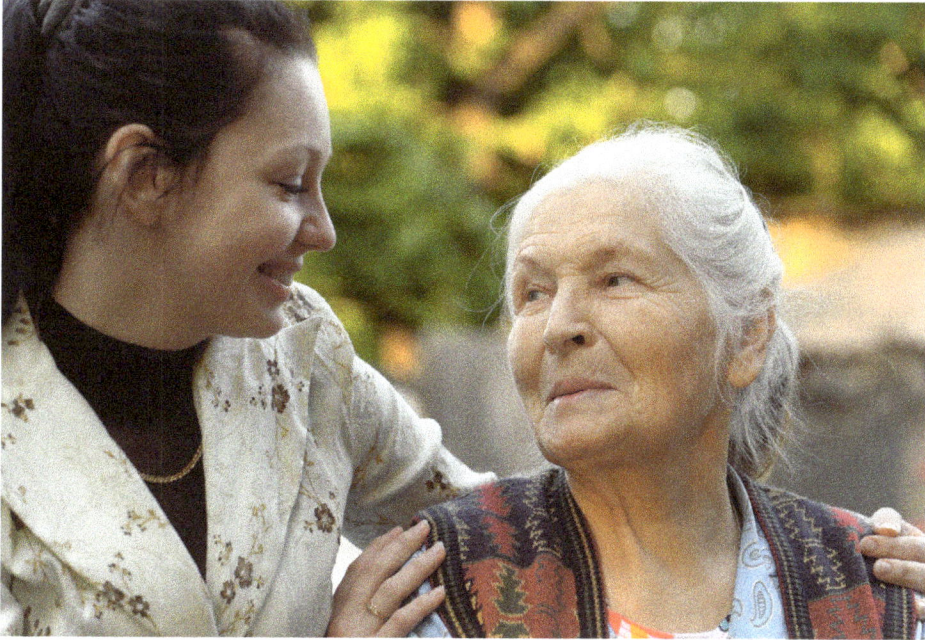

"Look here, doll. You don't know my story, but here goes! I hope you're ready for this." Dee grins at me over tea and a batch of homemade chocolate-chip-and-oatmeal cookies I had brought. I met with Deborah Huntington, a fiery 92-year-old with a sweet tooth and sharp tongue, to conduct this reminiscence interview. Her grandparents belonged to the original Higginbotham clan from the county of Cheshire, England, who arrived on the U.S. East Coast in 1896. Her mother and father met and were married in Baltimore, Maryland, where Dee was born as the younger of two kids. Dee speaks English and a little bit of German, having worked as a secretary and librarian throughout her professional life. She is widowed with two daughters: Patti lives on the East Coast, but her other daughter, Laura, lives locally in Santa Rosa with Dee's only granddaughter, Kimberly.

---

* Note: This interview was an assignment as part of a Geriatric Foundations course. The course is taken in the sophomore year of a pre-licensure nursing program. Students were given guidelines for the interview. They were asked to interview adults 65 years of age or older, with their permission and without using any identifying information. Names in this essay were changed to protect identities. This face-to-face interview has not been altered or modified in any way. Permission was obtained to use this interview for learning purposes.

Childhood

When I ask Dee about her childhood, she describes herself as a tomboy. She played tennis and ran in school competitions, where her mother would cheer on the sidelines as her "biggest fan." Her mom wasn't as supportive of her recreational sports hobbies: Dee would come home covered in dirt from playing tackle football with the boys. She quoted her mother: "What am I going to do with you, Dee? Whenever I see the boys piled up on the floor, you're always at the bottom of the heap!" Her father only shook his head when he heard of Dee's antics. Her grandpa, or Pop, would say, "Let her be! Dee, you're a little fireball. You just keep on keepin' on."

As a child, Dee cherished her relationship with her grandparents; Pop owned a farm about two miles away from her house. She and her sister, Sarah, would ride their bikes together to visit their grandpa and grandma. The farm was her "second home"—"I was a hay-baler ... the sun shining, the fresh aroma of the green, green grass ... I loved being out there, especially in the summer with my Pop and Gramma." Dee noted that it was Pop and Gramma who taught her how to read. "I was always a lover of books; I learned to read at an early age ... It all started with comic books and a strawberry blonde detective named Nancy Drew." I confessed that Nancy Drew was the gateway book series to my own love with literature; the crime-solving teenager's impact had spanned from the 1930s to even my generation! In turn, Dee disclosed that she catalogued her comic book collection as a child. If her friends wanted to borrow a book, they would have to "check them out" and return them by the given due date. If it wasn't returned, Dee would get on her bicycle to collect a 5-cent fee! "That way I could buy a new comic book with the money. It was a great system."

During the War

During WWII, Dee worked comfortably as a secretary in an Annapolis office. Eventually they began enlisting the secretaries to help out naval officers. A "Captain Fowler" came in while Dee was typing away. She gasped upon seeing a "gigantic bear of a man" surveying the room. Her supervisor followed to call her and another secretary into the back office to say that Captain Fowler wanted the both of them to work for him. Dee asked, "What if I don't want to work with him?" Her supervisor replied that "No one says no to the Captain," so off to Captain Fowler's headquarters she went. She remembers the day she "broke the ice between [herself] and the Cap'n": One morning, a heavy calendar fell off the wall in Dee's office. The sound made her jump, it was so loud. Almost instantly, the captain's voice boomed through the walls, " DOLOREEEEEEES?! GET IN HERE!" Dee took her time walking over to the Captain's room, telling me she "wasn't scared of 'im." When asked what happened, she replied indignantly, "Your damn calendar fell off the wall." The captain pushed his chair back slowly, eyeing Dee carefully. He threw his head back, exploding into roaring laughter. "Afterward, I could do no wrong, Christina. We got along swimmingly. His wife pulled me aside once saying that 'he saw me like a daughter.'" In a singsong-y voice, Dee told me, "Per-son-a-li-ty! That always does it!" I couldn't help but nod, and shimmy with her, in agreement.

"Even though the war was going on, I had the time of my life during my twenties. All my friends were around Annapolis at the time, and I met my husband-to-be, Ron, at this time." Ron was a naval officer who worked under the Cap'n. "I looked up from my typewriter one day to see this handsome man in uniform staring at me, then gazing down to my legs. I was just … appalled. I'd never had anybody just so blatant. But I was downright flattered too!" Dee relayed that on their first date, Ron took her out for dinner and dancing, and eventually they went "steady." "He asked me if I would marry him and I said, 'Yes!'" They eventually settled down in the District of Colombia, where they stayed for 30 years.

Living in the District of Columbia

While living for those 30 years in Washington, D.C., Dee worked as a librarian at the Library of Congress. In reflecting on her job, she said her favorite years were when she worked at the Young Readers Center in the Thomas Jefferson Building. "Working with children was wonderful," she relayed. "To see their innocence, their silliness, preserved at that age!" Her two loves, "besides Ron and the kids," are people and books, so the job was a perfect fit for Dee. She had flexible enough hours to pick up her two kids from school and could be at home to share dinner at the family table. "It was important to me that the family eat together every night, no matter how busy we were."

Even as a mother, Dee still showcased her clever, "fireball" antics. "Ron and I sent the girls to parochial school, where I volunteered to drive the nuns around on errands." Dee described the one time they were stuck coming out of an alley for twenty minutes: "Traffic was so bad in D.C." Dee's creative mind flashed a light bulb: "I knew anybody would stop for a nun, so I asked Sister Grace to get out onto the street to direct traffic." And, lo and behold, Sister Grace's "blessed presence on the street" allowed for Dee to get the nuns home before dinner. Dee is still giddy, reflecting on that day: "Yippee!" Her joy in that "yippee" was such a pleasure to experience, and the story revealed Dee's cleverness to me even more. She went on, "I felt like I had outsmarted the Fates. Even better, Ron sported a look of horror that morphed into a 100-watt grin when I told him at dinner that night."

Retirement

Dee and Ron sported those 100-watt grins with each other even through retirement. Dee recounts their European tour, their first adventure as a retired couple. They traveled through Italy, Rome, Scotland, England, Germany, and Ireland together.

When asked about the highlights of her European tour, she told me her favorite country they visited was Ireland. With acres of spanning green dunes and beautiful coastlines, the Emerald Isle "captured [her] heart instantly." Dee reminisced over the epic golf adventure she and Ron shared—golfing was a pastime and passion of theirs. Dee playfully adopted an Irish accent: "Over wild and tumbling terrain between dunes and stirring sea, Ron and I played 18 holes near the Cliffs of Moher. I had never had more fun with a lad!"

Dee and I spoke more about her lad and about how it was to be widowed after decades of marriage. Ron was diagnosed with bowel cancer after a visit to the doctor upon finding blood in his stool. Dee relayed to me that Ron did not want a colostomy bag or any cancer treatment. He didn't want that life; he thought "death was inevitable" and didn't see the point in fighting cancer to the point where he would become "a shadow of a man." Dee continued, "Ron didn't want me to take care of him … cleaning up after him as he 'disintegrated to dust.'" I asked Dee if she let Ron have his way without a fight; did he not want more time? What about their retired life together? Dee told me that of course they fought about it. "But I understood that he didn't want to live life with such a great loss of dignity. And he didn't want me … and our children and grandchildren … to watch as it happened to him." I asked Dee what her greatest concern was when they learned of Ron's diagnosis, and she replied, "Losing him. That was my biggest fear. And I eventually did … but it was his time."

Ron was Dee's best friend, and she considered every day with him an adventure, even in the last days. When asked to describe her marriage, she stated, "We had a long, strong marriage of 52 years." My mouth agape in sheer appreciation, I congratulated her. They had passed even the golden anniversary! When I asked her what kind of relationship advice she would have for me, she said, "Be good. Be compassionate. Be kind to each other. Go slow." I asked, "Go slow?" and she replied, "It's not a marathon, doll. It's a … it's just a stroll."

Reflection

It was a wonderful opportunity to sit down with Dee while she reminisced on her life. Taking time to listen to someone's story is so worthwhile, and the interview provided a therapeutic outlet for her. She told me that speaking with me alleviated some stress, "an unidentifiable antsy-ness" she sometimes suffered. I felt that it also allowed her to further come to terms with her age and to be reminded of her appreciation for her life and experiences.

Dee was a fantastic storyteller! The way she told stories—or parables, rather—reminded me of my grandmother, Lola Topy. Thanks to my Lola Topy's influence, I was able to fill in the lyrics when Dee would break out into song whenever the mood struck her during the interview. The songs wouldn't be easily recognizable to someone from my generation otherwise! The songs we sang back and forth included "Moon River" and "I've Got the World on a String." With songs and stories, it felt so easy to connect with Dee. Further, we share a love of books and music and possess almost identical senses of humor.

I was blown away that at 92 years old, Dee bears no signs of dementia or any cognitive deficits whatsoever. It shows the power of keeping the adult mind active and engaged. Her many years as a librarian and her continued status as an avid reader contribute to that, as she reads the newspaper daily and always keeps a stack of novels on her nightstand.

I have so much admiration for this woman. She taught me so much in only a few hours of conversation. Each story revealed more and more of Dee's vivacious personality and the great wisdom she has to share. One statement she made that struck me was that she's "never met a stranger." I believe it; she thoroughly enjoys the presence of people and is so open to intellectual discussion and learning. Her life has been filled with many happy experiences but also heart-wrenching ones. Yet she shows no fear of the future. She "never let[s] the past defeat" her and always has a 100-watt grin and witty comment at the ready. Even at 92, Dee is a force to be reckoned with, bearing a personality and attitude toward life that I hope to emulate.

References

Administration for Community Living (ACL). (2024). *2023 profile of older Americans.* ACL. https://acl.gov/sites/default/files/Profile%20of%20OA/ACL_ProfileOlderAmericans 2023_508.pdf

American Psychological Association (APA). (2024). *Introduction to mentoring: A guide for mentors and mentees.* https://www.apa.org/education-career/grad/mentoring

Australian Human Rights Commission (AHRC). (2021). *Employing and retaining older workers.* https://humanrights.gov.au/sites/default/files/document/publication/ahri_employingolder-workers_april_2021.pdf

Cavatore, M., Stovell, J., & Williamson, C. (2021). *Voice training: A facilitator's guide.* HelpAge International. https://www.helpage.org/silo/files/voice-training-a-facilitators-guide.pdf

Centers for Disease Control (CDC). (2024a, March). *About productive aging and work.* National Institute for Occupational Safety and Health (NIOSH). https://www.cdc.gov/niosh/aging/about/index.html#cdc_health_safety_special_topic_risks-health-safety-and-aging

Centers for Disease Control (CDC). (2024b, March). *Data and statistics on aging workers.* National Institute for Occupational Safety and Health (NIOSH). https://www.cdc.gov/niosh/aging/data-research/

Fiske, S. T., & Becker, T. (Eds.). (2022). *Understanding the aging workforce: Defining a research agenda.* The National Academies Press. https://doi.org/10.17226/26173

Fry, R., & Braga, D. (2023, December). *Older workers are growing in number and earning higher wages.* Pew Research Center. https://www.pewresearch.org/social-trends/2023/12/14/older-workers-are-growing-in-number-and-earning-higher-wages/

Mahler, C. (2021 August 4). *United Nations General Assembly Human Rights Council, report of the independent expert on the enjoyment of all human rights by older persons,* United Nations. https://digitallibrary.un.org/record/3938306?ln=en&v=pdf

Phoenix, C. (2020). *Campaigning to tackle ageism: Current practices and suggestions for moving forward.* World Health Organization. https://www.who.int/publications/m/item/campaigning-to-tackle-ageism

UNITAR Division for People and Social Inclusion. (2023). *2nd round: Access to justice for older persons Effective and participative systems* [Video]. YouTube. https://www.youtube.com/watch?v=Tgvp8XZGZkY

UNITAR Division for People and Social Inclusion. (2024, July4). *Mainstreaming knowledge on ageing* [Videos]. YouTube. https://www.youtube.com/playlist?list=PLQR8YH-

United Nations. (n.d.). *Four action areas and four "enablers," with older people at the centre* [Video]. U.N. Decade of Healthy Ageing: The Platform. https://www.decadeofhealthyageing.org/about/about-us/what-is-the-decade

United Nations Human Rights Council (UNHRC). (October 14, 2021). *Human rights of older YtQS9wxqOw4udFejL5q5SMMowD persons.* Resolution adopted by the Human Rights Council on 7 October 2021. https://undocs.org/+A/HRC/RES 48/3

United States Department of Health and Human Services (USDHHS). (n.d.-a). *Healthy people 2030 framework.* Office of Disease Prevention and Health Promotion https://health.gov/healthypeople/about/healthy-people-2030-framework

U.S. Department of Health and Human Services (USDHHS). (n.d.-b). *ODPHP healthy aging custom list.* Office of Disease Prevention and Health Promotion. https://health.gov/healthypeople/custom-list?list=odphps-healthy-aging-custom-list

United States Department of Health and Human Services (USDHHS). (n.d.-c). *Reduce fall-related deaths among older adults—IVP-08.* Office of Disease Prevention and Health Promotion. https://health.gov/healthypeople/objectives-and-data/browse-objectives/injury-prevention/reduce-fall-related-deaths-among-older-adults-ivp-08

World Health Organization (WHO). (2021a). *Global campaign to combat ageism-toolkit: Initiating a conversation about ageism* [PowerPoint slides]. https://www.who.int/publications/m/item/global-campaign-to-combat-ageism-toolkit

World Health Organization (WHO). (2021b). *Global report on ageism.* https://www.who.int/publications/i/item/9789240016866

World Health Organization (WHO). (2024). *Making older persons visible in the Sustainable Development Goals' monitoring framework and indicators.* https://www.who.int/publications/i/item/9789240090248

Selected Bibliography

Amankwah, F., Alper, J., & Nass, S. J. (2024). *Unequal treatment revisited: The current state of racial and ethnic disparities in health care: Proceedings of a workshop.* The National Academies Press. https://doi.org/10.17226/27448

Beauchamp, M., Hao, Q., Kuspinar, A., Alder, G., Makino, K., Nouredanesh, M., Zhao, Y., Mikton, C., Thiyagarajan, J. A., Diaz, T., & Raina, P. (2023). Measures of perceived mobility ability in community-dwelling older adults: A systematic review of psychometric properties. *Age and Ageing, 52*(4), iv100–iv111. https://doi.org/10.1093/ageing/afad124

Beauchamp, M. K, Hao, Q., Kuspinar, A., Thiyagarajan, J. A., Mikton, C., Diaz, T., & Raina, P. (2023). A unified framework for the measurement of mobility in older persons, *Age and Ageing, 52*(4), iv82–iv85. https://doi.org/10.1093/ageing/afad125

Benjamin, G. C., DeVoe, J. E., Amankwah, F. K., & Nass, S. J. (2024). *Ending unequal treatment: Strategies to achieve equitable health care and optimal health for all.* The National Academies Press. https://doi.org/10.17226/27820

Bentley, T., Onnis, L.-A., Vasilley, A., Farr-Wharton, B., Caponecchia, C., Andrew, C., O'Neill, S., De Almeida Neto, A., Huron, V., & Green, N. (2023). A systematic review of literature on occupational health and safety for older workers. *Ergonomics, 66*(12), 1968–1983, https://doi.org/10.1080/00140139.2023.2176550

Burke, S. P., Polsky, D. E., & Geller, A. B. (2023). *Federal policy to advance racial, ethnic, and tribal health equity.* The National Academies Press. https://doi.org/10.17226/26834.

Canopy—A Social Imagination Project. (2021). *Talk about ageism with birthday cards* [Video]. YouTube. https://www.youtube.com/watch?v=NVHrgNfEXKM

Chadha, S., Dillard, L. K., Mariotti, S. P., & Keel, S. (2023). Monitoring hearing and vision functions in older adults: rationale and process. *Age and Ageing, 52*(4), iv158–iv161. https://doi.org/10.1093/ageing/afad123

Chin, M. H., Afsar-Manesh, N., Bierman, A. S., Chang, C., Colon-Rodriguez, C. J., Dullabh, P., Duran, D. G., Fair, M., Hernandez-Boussard, T. Hightower, M., Jain., A., Jordan, W. B., Konya, S., Moore, R. H., Moore, T. T., Rodriguez, R., Shaheen, G., Snyder, L. P., Srinivasan, M., Umscheid, C. A., & Ohno-Machado, L. (2023). Guiding principles to address the impact of algorithm bias on racial and ethnic disparities in health and health care. *JAMA Network Open, 6*(12): e2345050. https://doi:10.1001/jamanetworkopen.2023.46050

Crist, M. Appiah, G., Leidel, L., & Stoney, R. (2024). *Medical tourism CDC yellow book 2024, traveler's health.* CDC. https://wwwnc.cdc.gov/travel/yellowbook/2024/health-care-abroad/medical-tourism

De Looze, C., Feeney, J., Seeher, K. M., Thiyagarajan, J. A., Diaz, T., & Kenny, R. A. (2023). Assessing cognitive function in longitudinal studies of ageing worldwide: Some practical considerations. *Age and Ageing, 52*(4), iv13–iv25. https://doi.org/10.1093/ageing/afad122

Doing Good Together. (2024). *14 inspiring picture books to celebrate seniors and embrace ageing.* https://www.doinggoodtogether.org/bhf-book-lists/picture-books-about-aging

Evans, K. N., Martinez, O., King, H., Van Den Berg J. J., Fields, E. L., Lanier, Y., Hussen, S. A., Malave-Rivera, S. M., Duncan, D. T., Gaul, Z., & Buchacz, K. (2023). Utilizing community based participatory research methods in Black/African American and Hispanic/Latinx communities in the U.S.: The CDC minority HIV research initiative (MARI-round 4). *Journal of Community Health, 48,* 698–710. https://doi.org/10.1007/s10900-023-01209-5

Gichu, M., & Harwood, R. H. (2023). Measurement of healthy ageing. *Age and Ageing, 52*(4), iv3–iv5. https://doi.org/10.1093/ageing/afad118

Gignac, M. A. M., Bowring, J., Shahidi, F. V., Kristman, V., Cameron, J. I., & Jetha, A. (2024). Workplace disclosure decisions of older workers wanting to remain employed: A qualitative study of factors considered when contemplating revealing or concealing support needs. *Work, Aging, and Retirement, 10,* 174–187. https://doi.org/10.1093/workar/waac029

UN Decade of Healthy Ageing. (2021). *Global campaign to combat ageism—#AWorld4AllAges* [Video]. YouTube. https://www.youtube.com/watch?v=7tThSqTWsCs

Gutiérrez-Robledo, L. M., Tella-Vega, P. García-Chanes, R. E., Lozano-Juárez, L. R., Medina-Campos, R. H., García-Andrade, S., Escamilla-Núñez, A., Thiyagarajan, J. A., Diaz, T., Mikton, C., & García-Peña, C. (2023). Psychometric properties of ability to contribute measurements as a domain of functional ability of older persons: A COSMIN systematic review. *Age and Ageing, 52*(4), iv138–iv148. https://doi.org/10.1093/ageing/afad099

Han, E.-J., Han, Z.-A., Kim, H., & Jung, T. R. (2023). Monitoring healthy ageing for the next decade: South Korea's perspective. *Age and Ageing, 52*(4), iv10–iv12. https://doi.org/10.1093/ageing/afad102

HelpAge International. (2021). *Exposing systemic ageism* [Video]. YouTube. https://www.youtube.com/watch?v=ZwrZ3Da6q64

HelpAge International. (2016). *Ageism is all around us—Hear how it affects people all around the world* [Video]. YouTube. https://www.youtube.com/watch?v=sv41CdxImiU

Honvo, G., Sabico, S., Veronese, N., Bruyère, O., Rizzoli, R., Thiyagarajan, J. A., Mikton, C., Diaz, T., Cooper, C., & Reginster, J.-Y. (2023). Measures of attributes of locomotor capacity in older people: a systematic literature review following the COSMIN methodology. *Age and Ageing, 52*(4), iv44–iv66. https://doi.org/10.1093/ageing/afad139

Institute for Health Metrics and Evaluation-Centre for Global Health Inequalities Research (IHME-CHAIN Collaborators). (2024). Effects of education on adult mortality: A global systematic review and meta-analysis. *The Lancet, 9*(155–165). https://doi.org/10.1016/S2468-2667(23)00306-7

Irving, P., Kramer, B., Kung, J., & Frauenheim, E. (2022). 7 principles to attract and retain older frontline workers. *Harvard Business Review.* https://hbr.org/2022/12/7-principles-to-attract-and-retain-older-frontline-workers

Julião, P. L., Fernandes, O. B., Alves, J. P., Thiyagarajan, J. A., Mikton, C., Diaz, T., & Pais, S. (2023). A systematic review of reviews on the psychometric properties of measures of older persons' ability to build and maintain social relationships. *Age and Ageing, 52*(4) iv133–iv137. https://doi.org/10.1093/ageing/afad106

Knoop, V., Mathot, E., Louter, F., Beckwee, D., Mikton, C., Diaz, T., Thiyagarajan, J. A., & Bautmans, I. (2023). Measurement properties of instruments to measure the fatigue domain of vitality capacity in community-dwelling older people: An umbrella review of systematic reviews and meta-analysis. *Age and Ageing, 52*(4), iv26–iv43. https://doi.org/10.1093/ageing/afad140

Kuspinar, A., Mehdipour, A., Beauchamp, M. A., Hao, Q., Cino, E., Mikton, C., Thiyagarajan, J. A., Diaz, T., & Raina, P. (2023). Assessing the measurement properties of life-space mobility measures in community-dwelling older adults: A systematic review. *Age and Ageing, 52*(4), iv86–iv99. https://doi.org/10.1093/ageing/afad119

Leigh, J.-H., Lee, H., Yoon, J., Han, E.-J., Park, E., Jung, T. R., Thiyagarajan, J. A., & Han, Z.-A. (2023). Effective service coverage of long-term care among older persons in South Korea. *Age and Ageing, 52*(4), iv162–iv169. https://doi.org/10.1093/ageing/afad120

Mansor, N., Awang, H., Thiyagarajan, J. A., Mikton, C., & Diaz, T. (2023). Measures of ability to learn, grow and make decisions among older persons: A systematic review of measurement properties. *Age and Ageing, 52*(4), iv118–iv132. https://doi.org/10.1093/ageing/afad101

McDonald, T. A. M., & Scudder, A. (2024). Mind the NIH-funding gap: Structural discrimination in physical health-related research for cognitively able autistic adults. *Journal of Autism and Developmental Disorders, 54*, 1411–1424. https://doi.org/10.1007/s10803-022-05856w

Murray, A. J., & De La Fuente-Núñez, V. (2023). Development of the item pool for the "WHO-ageism scale": conceptualisation, item generation and content validity assessment. *Age and Ageing, 52*(4), iv149–iv157. https://doi.org/10.1093/ageing/afad105

National Institute on Aging. (n.d.). National Institutes of Health. https://www.nia.nih.gov/

Nissim, N. R., Fudge, M. R., Lachner, C., Lucas, J. A., Graff-Radford, N. R., & Day, G. S. (2023). Age-specific barriers and facilitators to research participation among underrepresented African Americans. *Alzheimer's & Dementia, 16*(S22), e073810

Oster, C., Hines, S., Rissel, C., Asante, D., Khadka, J., Seeher, K. M., Thiyagarajan, J. A., Mikton, C., Diaz, T., & Isaac, V. (2023). A systematic review of the measurement properties of aspects of psychological capacity in older adults. *Age and Ageing, 52*(4), iv67–iv81. https://doi.org/10.1093/ageing/afad100

PBS. (2023). Superagers: Getting old, living young [Video]. https://www.pbs.org/video/superagers-getting-old-living-young-bx7wti/

Smart, M. (2021). *10 positive picture books about senior citizens and aging.* https://mayasmart.com/10-positive-picture-books-about-senior-citizens-and-aging/

Tamlyn, B. A., Tjilos, M., Bosch, N. A., Barnett, K. G., Perkins, R. B., Walkey, M. D., Assoumou, S. A., Linas, B. P., Drainoni, M.-L. (2023). At the intersection of trust and mistrust: A qualitative analysis of motivators and barriers to research participation at a safety-net hospital. *Health Expectations, 26,* 1118–1126. https://doi.org/10.1111/hex.13726

Taylor, M. (2024), *Children's books about memory loss, aging, and Alzheimer's.* Imagination Soup. https://imaginationsoup.net/childrens-books-aging-memory-loss-alzheimers/

U.S. Department of Justice, Civil Rights Division. (n.d.). *Mobility devices.* https://www.ada.gov/topics/mobility-devices/

U.S. Department of Justice, Civil Rights Division. (2010). *ADA standards for accessible design.* https://www.ada.gov/law-and-regs/design-standards/

U.S. Department of Justice, Civil Rights Division. (2012, March 8). *Americans with disabilities act title III regulations.* https://www.ada.gov/law-and-regs/regulations/title-iii-regulations/

U.S. Department of Justice, Civil Rights Division. (2022, May 12). *Algorithms, artificial intelligence, and disability discrimination in hiring.* https://www.ada.gov/resources/ai-guidance/

U.S. Department of Justice, Civil Rights Division. (2024, April 8). *Fact sheet: New rule on the accessibility of web content and mobile apps provided by state and local governments.* https://www.ada.gov/resources/2024-03-08-web-rule/

U.S. Department of Justice, Office of Public Affairs. (2024, July 26). *Justice Department to publish final rule to improve access to medical care for people with disabilities* [Press release]. https://www.justice.gov/opa/pr/justice-department-publish-final-rule-improve-access-medical-care-people-disabilities

U.S. Department of Labor, Occupational Safety and Health Administration. (n.d.). https://www.osha.gov/

U.S. Department of State, Bureau of Consular Affairs. (n.d.). Your Health Abroad, International Travel. https://travel.state.gov/content/travel/en/international-travel/before-you-go/your-health-abroad.html

Venkatapuram, S., & Thiyagarajan, J. A. (2023). The capability approach and the WHO healthy ageing framework (for the UN Decade of Healthy Ageing). *Age and Ageing, 52*(4) iv6–iv9. https://doi.org/10.1093/ageing/afad126

Williams, T., Geffen, L., Kalula, S., Stein, D. J., Thiyagarajan, J. A., Mikton, C., & Diaz, T. (2023). A systematic review of measures of ability to meet basic needs in older persons. *Age and Ageing, 52*(4), iv112–iv11. https://doi.org/10.1093/ageing/afad121

World Health Organization (WHO). (n.d.). *Maternal, newborn, child and adolescent health and ageing data portal: Ageing data.* Data Platform. https://platform.who.int/data/maternal-newborn-child-adolescent-ageing/ageing-data

Websites

INDEX

www.ingramcontent.com/pod-product-compliance
Lightning Source LLC
Chambersburg PA
CBHW061417210326
41598CB00035B/6246